DEPRESSION

Edited by **Dagmar Breznoščáková**

Depression
http://dx.doi.org/10.5772/63698
Edited by Dagmar Breznoščáková

Contributors
Azizuddin Khan, Danielle Danielle Pereira, Noboru Motomura, Yuko Okamoto, Elena V. Bouzinova, Sofie Laage Christiansen, Hovhannes M Manvelyan, Aleksandra Karapetyan, Yasemin Yavuzer, Zeynep Karataş, Hong Yao, Xiaowen Ji, Lai Wan Chan, Celia Hoi Yan Chan

Published by InTech
Janeza Trdine 9, 51000 Rijeka, Croatia

Publishing Process Manager Iva Simcic
Technical Editor SPi Global
Cover InTech Design team

First published March, 2017
Printed in Croatia
Legal deposit, Croatia: National and University Library in Zagreb

Additional hard copies can be obtained from orders@intechopen.com

Depression, Edited by Dagmar Breznoščáková
p. cm.
Print ISBN 978-953-51-3059-8
Online ISBN 978-953-51-3060-4

For EU product safety concerns:
IN TECH d.o.o., Prolaz Marije Krucifikse Kozulić 3, 51000 Rijeka, Croatia,
info@intechopen.com or visit our website at intechopen.com.

Meet the editor

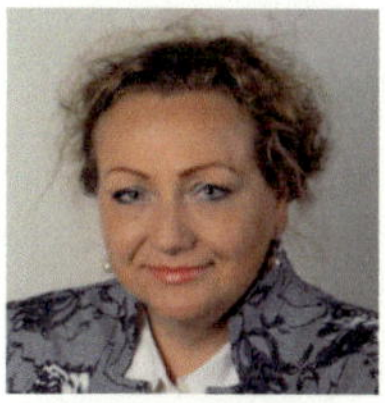

Since 2016, Dagmar Breznoščáková, MD, PhD, has been the vice-president of Slovak Psychiatric Association and CPT member of the Council of Europe with respect to Slovak Republic. Since 2012, she has been the chairwoman of the Section of Psychopharmacology Slovak Psychiatric Association, Slovak Medical Association. In 2006, she was registered in the List of Experts of the Ministry of Justice SR and has since worked as an expert witness in psychiatry. Since 2006, she has also been engaging in private outpatient psychiatric care and psychotherapy. She successfully completed a 4.5-year European training in cognitive behavioral psychotherapy and completed her postgraduate studies at the Masaryk University in Brno, Czech Republic. The topic of her postgraduate study was "Carbohydrate Metabolism and Depression." After graduation, she started to work as a resident at the Department of Psychiatry, Faculty of Medicine, UPJŠ, and Faculty Hospital in Košice. Since 2005, she has been working as an assistant professor at the Faculty of Medicine, Faculty of Law and Philosophy UPJŠ in Košice. She also lectures and publishes in her field, focusing on affective and anxiety disorders, particularly bipolar disorder, comorbidity of mental disorders, and psychosomatic connections. She is a coauthor of several chapters in foreign as well as domestic publications and author of psychoeducational handbooks for patients and their relatives, all in all over 150 publication outputs. She holds prizes for the best original work for the journal of psychiatry practice and figures in the biographical encyclopedia of Slovak republic personalities Who Is Who. She organizes and actively participates in various psychoeducational and antistigma activities and is the chairwoman of ROZ ODOS Košice o. z., joining together patients, their relatives, professionals, as well as the general public or supporters.

Contents

Preface

Depressive disorders can be seen as a disturbance to the balance of mind and body. Because it is a mental disorder and psychiatry is a branch of medicine, the question how mind and body interact in depression should be treated as a medical rather than metaphysical mind-body problem. The relation between mind and body as it pertains to this illness should be construed in teleological rather than causal terms. Mental states like beliefs and emotions serve an adaptive purpose by constraining the physiologic systems involved in the body's stress response, thus preserving homeostasis and protecting us from various disorders. Depression results when the mind fails its constraining role.

In first Section in context of disturbed circadian rhythm, it is relevant to comment on the type of rhythmic abnormality. It is highly individual among depressed patients and may be expressed as a phase advance or phase delay of rhythms and/or increase or decrease in the amplitude. *Elena Bouzinova* and *Laage Christiansen* discuss the molecular mechanisms underlying rhythmic abnormalities in depression as results of studies performed on humans and using animal model of depression. Since the development of an anhedonic-like phenotype is associated with alterations in clock gene expression, a normalization of this pattern is likely to be essential for the recovery from the pathological state. *Danielle M. Pereira* and *Azizuddin Khan* discussed three major hypotheses regarding the lateralization of emotion in the brain —the right hemisphere hypothesis, the valence hypothesis, and the approach-withdrawal hypothesis. It has been found that persons with depression show left frontal hypoactivity and right frontal hyperactivity. The asymmetry may also be a biological marker of depression, with research evidence showing that it is found in remitted depressives and in infants of depressed mothers. Currently, research in this area focuses on identifying the mechanism underlying the link between the asymmetry and depression.

The prevalence of anxiety and depression of patients after cardiovascular surgeries has varied from 10% to 60% and has been likely higher than that of general people as is reported in second Section. From the limited studies about patients over 6 months after surgery, *Yuko Okamoto* and *Noboru Motomura* guessed the following about the trends of anxiety and depression of patients with CABG without any other additional intervention programs before/after surgery: (1) patients improved scores of anxiety and depression 3–6 months after surgery, (2) anxiety decreased considerably for about 6 months after CABG and then leveled out for some time, and (3) depression remained a bit higher 6 months and more after CABG. *Aleksandra A. Karapetyan* and *Hovhannes M. Manvelyan* talk about a vicious circle of pain and depression in which pain worsens symptoms of depression and then the resulting depression exacerbates feelings of pain. Fibromyalgia (FM) is one of most common chronic pain syndromes, affecting up to 5% of the world population; is characterized by diffuse widespread body pain, with defined tender points and clinical features; and also triggers development of depression. Depression severity in patients with fibromyalgia worsens severity of pain. These findings are consistent with the results of a number of authors: depressive disorders observed in approximately 90% of patients with FM. Pain triggers development of depressive conditions in patients with chronic character of pain; time-course of disease shows certain pattern of increase of severity of depression and worsens long-term outcomes. Patients with chronic pain must be necessarily evaluated for depression, and successful management of the pain severity in those patients must include treatment of depressive mood too.

Yasemin Yavuzer and *Zeynep Karatas,* in Section three, state that five variables (negative automatic thoughts, life satisfaction, number of symptoms, psychologizing, and normalizing) are significant predictors in explaining the depression level of young adults. Together, these five variables explain 52% of the young adults' depression. Another finding of the study is that negative automatic thoughts of young adults make them negatively assess quality of life, and this causes the depression levels to increase. Complex interaction among depression, sleep, and physical illnesses was highlighted by *Sylvia Hong Yao* and *colleagues* as the essential mind-body connection in the planning of integrative care and other clinical services. A number of eastern mind-body practices, such as Qigong, acupuncture, and meditation, have been frequently studied indicating the efficacy of mind-body connection in complementary therapies. They describe the Integrative Body-Mind-Spirit (I-BMS) group work, which has been found effective in addressing comorbid depressed mood and somatic afflictions, especially sleep disturbances.

This book is perhaps a small step in attempting to integrate a new synthesis of basic neurosciences, molecular and biological markers of depression via comorbidity, and clinical psychiatry in the sense of selected psychological aspects leading to development of possible depression.

Dagmar Breznoščáková, MD, PhD
First Department of Psychiatry, School of Medicine
University of P. J. Šafárik,
Košice, Slovakia

Section 1

Biological and Molecular Markers of Depression

Chapter 1

Clock Genes in Depression

Sofie Laage Christiansen and Elena V. Bouzinova

Additional information is available at the end of the chapter

http://dx.doi.org/10.5772/67261

Abstract

Data demonstrate that abnormal regulation of the circadian system can result in cardiovascular disease, metabolic syndrome, obesity, immune dysfunction, increased risk for cancer, reproductive complications, etc. It is highly individual among depressed patients and may be expressed as a phase advance or phase delay of rhythms and/or increase or decrease in the amplitude. The stress-induced anhedonic-like state characterizes by hypothermia, hypercortisolemia, and hypermelatoninemia associated with disturbances in the circadian system. Mainly Per2 and Bmal1 demonstrate altered expression in the brain and liver: expression of Per2 is sensitive to stress and changes in Bmal1 mostly associated with depressive behavior. The Per1 expression is sustainable in maintaining the circadian rhythm. A normalization of the expression patterns is likely to be essential for the recovery from the pathological state. Depression is a high prevalent disorder. The number of incidents is rising due to changes in lifestyle. The symptomatology is inconsistent and it is difficult to agree on one hypothesis. The disturbances of the 24 h circadian rhythm may be a factor in the development of major depressive disorder. The molecular biology underlying a causal relationship between circadian rhythm and mood disorders is slowly being unraveled. However, many questions still need to be answered.

Keywords: depression, anhedonia, diurnal rhythms, clock genes, phase markers, chronic mild stress

1. Hypothesis of disturbed circadian rhythms in depression: evidence in support of a dysfunction of the endogenous clock machinery in depression

For more than 40 decades, several lines of evidence have linked depression to disturbances of the circadian system. Abnormalities in the sleep pattern, such as early awakening in the morning hours, are found in up to 80% of the depressed patients [1]. Treatment with antidepressants can restore the chronobiological changes [2]. Work shift or jetlag (manipulations of the circadian rhythm) increases the risk of developing a depression [3]. Individuals born with a shifted or arrhythmic biological clock have a higher risk of becoming depressed [4]. Circadian manipulations, such as bright light therapy and total sleep deprivation, are capable to reverse depressive symptoms within hours [2, 5]. The severity of the depressive symptoms follows a 24 h rhythm most dominant in the morning [6]. Blunted or abnormal circadian rhythm of temperature and hormone secretion is a prominent feature in depressed people. Also, depressed individuals elicit altered brain and locomotor activity [7]. Decreased hippocampal neurogenesis is found in depressed patients [8], and neurogenesis is under the control of the so-called clock genes (clock genes are making up the biological clock of the body) [9]. Clock gene polymorphism has been found to be associated with mood disorders [10]. Involvement of the circadian system in depression is emphasized by the seasonal affective disorder (SAD), a subtype of depression also called winter depression. SAD is defined as recurrent episodes of depression in the autumn and winter [11]. It is shown that SAD is more common in areas of the world receiving less sunlight [12]. The late chronotype/eveningness is associated with increased risk of developing a depression compared to the early chronotype/morningness [13]. Treatment with a third-generation antidepressant, agomelatine, is known to act through the recovery of the disturbed circadian rhythm [14].

Besides the involvement of the circadian system in depression, disturbances of the 24 h rhythm also possess a major risk to health in general [15]. Abnormal regulation of the circadian system can result in cardiovascular disease, metabolic syndrome, obesity, immune dysfunction, increased risk for cancer, and reproductive complications [16].

In the context of a disturbed circadian rhythm, it is also relevant to comment on the possible types of rhythmic abnormalities, which are highly individual among depressed patients. The circadian rhythm abnormalities may be expressed as a phase advance or a phase delay of rhythms and/or increase or decrease in the amplitude [17].

2. Introduction to circadian rhythms

So, what is a circadian rhythm exactly?

The word circadian is derived from Latin and means *about a day*. The most prominent circadian rhythm is the sleep/wake cycle, but most physiological and behavioral processes of the body follow a 24 h rhythm, such as activity, core body temperature, hormone levels, cognition, attention, and even mood [18].

One of the most essential time givers or zeitgebers (ZTs) is the light since it has the ability to entrain the organism to the 24 h circadian day [19]. Entraining information reaches the master clock of the body, the suprachiasmatic nucleus (SCN), via the retinohypothalamic tract [20] (**Figure 1A**). The SCN neurons project to multiple areas in the brain (for a review, see [21]). However, the paraventricular nucleus (PVN) of the hypothalamus and the pineal gland are the major SCN output [22].

Before presenting the mechanism of the molecular clock, two core hormones, melatonin and cortisol (corticosterone in rodents), of the circadian system deserve attention.

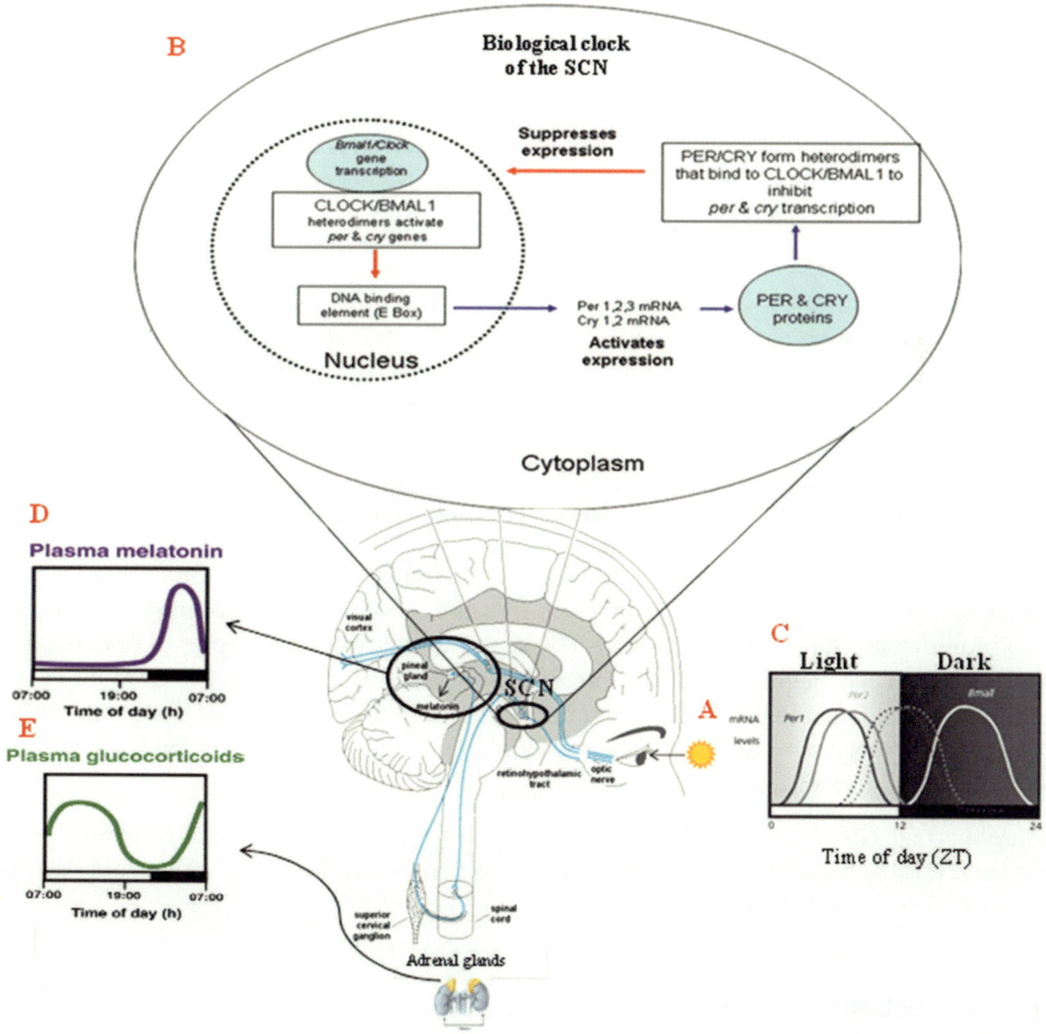

Figure 1. Essential components of the human circadian system. (A) Light and dark cues are the strongest zeitgebers of the circadian rhythm. The light sends photic information to the retina, which is the inner and light-sensitive layer of the eye. Through the optic nerve, the signal reaches the brain. A projection innervates the master clock, the SCN, via the retinohypothalamic tract that is anatomically and functionally different from the other neural pathways that reach the visual cortex. (B) Positive and negative feedback loop of the clock genes organizes the biological clock of the SCN. (C) Through rhythmic expression of the clock genes (light-sensitive genes have been selected as an example), the circadian rhythm is resynchronized every day. (D) From the SCN, a multisynaptic pathway leads to the pineal gland, where melatonin is secreted in the rhythmic manner as a signal of darkness. Entraining cues also affect the adrenal gland, which secretes corticosterone. (E) The maximum of corticosterone secretion occurs in the morning and associated with awakening. Modified from Refs. [120–122].

2.1. The role of melatonin in the development of depression with focus on the circadian rhythm

Melatonin is a hormone under direct control of the SCN and is one of the most important players in resetting the circadian rhythm every day [23]. It is primarily secreted from the pineal gland and mainly synthesized at night in all species [24] (**Figure 1D**). Due to minor sensitivity to the environment, melatonin is a stable marker of the circadian phase [25]. In humans, the circadian phase is determined by measuring the onset of melatonin secretion by dim light in the evening, the so-called dim light melatonin onset (DLMO). Thus, from 18:00 until prior to bedtime, the concentration of plasma melatonin is measured every 30 min [26]. The DLMO was first used in the 1980s [27], and today it is acknowledged as one of the best markers of the phase [28].

Since the 1980s, melatonin has been linked to depression, and low melatonin levels have been observed in depressed patients [29, 30]. Since serotonin is the precursor of melatonin, the low levels of melatonin can partly be explained by the low serotonin level found in some depressed individuals [31]. In contrast, other studies have reported elevated levels of melatonin during depression [32, 33]. Finally, a phase shift in the secretion of melatonin has been linked to depression [34].

2.2. The role of cortisol in depression with focus on the circadian rhythm

Cortisol is an important element for maintaining the daily circadian rhythm. The secretion of cortisol is associated with awakening and increases shortly after awakening: the cortisol awakening response (CAR) [35] (**Figure 1E**). A rise in the early morning level of cortisol is stated to be a reliable marker of the adrenocortical activity if measured repeatedly at the time of awakening. The lowest concentration is found in the beginning of the evening [36]. Compared to melatonin cortisol is a less robust phase marker since its secretion is affected by environmental factors, most importantly stress.

An abnormal circadian rhythm of cortisol is well described in a subgroup of depressed patients. Also, a blunted circadian rhythm [37] and an elevated level of cortisol are specific features of depressed individuals [38].

3. The mechanism of the molecular clock

The internal biological clock or the master clock is believed to hierarchically control all circadian rhythms in the body. It is located deep inside the brain in the anterior part of the hypothalamus and named by its location, the SCN [39]. The SCN is built up from the positive and negative feedback loops of so-called clock genes. Some of the most essential clock genes are the period genes (*Per*) 1–3, bone and muscle ARNT-like 1 (*Bmal1*), circadian locomotor output cycle caput (*Clock*), and the cryptochrome (*Cry*) 1–2. However, the clock genes are not exclusive components of the clockwork. Other well-known signaling proteins and cytosolic factors have been revealed as important players of the circadian machinery. Briefly, the main regulatory unit of the clock genes, a heterodimeric complex of CLOCK and BMAL1, is formed in the cytoplasm and translocated to the cell nucleus. In the nucleus, the dimer binds to an e-box motif and drives the transcription of the *Per* and *Cry* genes. These genes are translated into the corresponding protein products, and like the BMAL1 and CLOCK, they dimerize, enter the nucleus, and interfere with the BMAL1/CLOCK complex, thus inhibiting its transcription. For a review, see [40] (**Figure 1B**). This so-called cycle of gene activation and inhibition is self-sustained and takes about 24 h [41]. The expression of *Per1* and *Per2* genes is the light-sensitive elements of the cycle. Hence expression starts by light activation and reaches peak level at noon. The protein product reaches peak level approximately 6 h later (**Figure 1C**).

It is a well-known fact that the clock genes are not only found in the SCN machinery, but in most central regions [42] and peripheral tissues, including the heart and liver [43–46]. A functional molecular clock is even observed in cell cultures [47]. Food is the strongest cue able to entrain peripheral clocks without affecting the SCN rhythm [48], but social activity and locomotor activity are also known to synchronize the phase [49].

4. The clock genes in major depression

Implications of the circadian system in depression have gained much attention in recent years. However, the biology underlying the association or causal relationship between circadian rhythm and mood disorders is still mostly unknown, and no clock genes specific for the disease have been convincingly identified yet.

In particular, in the late 1990s, the clock genes gained increased awareness due to important breakthroughs in the understanding of the molecular clock [18]. The following quote is from Science (December, 1998):

"Nineteenth-century philosophers proposed that God was a clockmaker who created the world and let it run. Modern biologists might in part agree, for it's clear that evolution has carefully crafted clocks that allow almost all organisms to follow the rhythm of the sun. In 1998, a volley of rapid-fire discoveries revealed the stunning universality of the clock workings. Across the tree of life, from bacteria to humans, clocks use oscillating levels of proteins in feedback loops to keep time. Perhaps more amazing, fruit flies and mice—separated by nearly 700 million years of evolution—share the very same timekeeping proteins. Now that they better understand the cellular clock, scientists can begin to manipulate it, with applications from curing jet lag to brightening winter depression."[1]

Two studies, published in 2012 and 2013, demonstrate the implication of dysfunction of clock genes in human depression [50, 51]. The later work is most convincing. Li and coworkers used transcriptome-wide analysis on high-quality postmortem brain tissue and showed that several hundred transcripts in six selected structures of the human brain had 24 h rhythmic-

[1]http://science.sciencemag.org/content/282/5397/news-summaries

ity. Most interestingly, they measured a much weaker 24 h rhythm in the brains of depressed patients and postulated that it could be a consequence of a shift in peak and a dislocated phase relationships between different clock genes. Sequeira and coworkers report a reduced *Per1* expression at one time point in postmortem brain tissue from depressed suicide individuals compared to non-suicide depressed individuals, indicating for the first time the association between the clock genes and depression [50].

Few other studies also report abnormal clock gene expression in the human brain, but not in relation to depression [52, 53].

In general, postmortem studies are challenged by difficulties related to the differences in the precise time of death, which is of great importance in the studies of the clock genes. Furthermore, the length of the postmortem interval is a potential confound in all studies [54].

The involvement of the clock genes in depression is also evident from several genetic studies. Polymorphisms of clock genes have been reported in depressed patients [55–59]. Despite the number of studies investigating the polymorphism in clock genes, the validity of the studies might be discussed due to small sample size and low reproducibility [60].

5. The clock genes in animal models of depression

Most studies on clock genes have been conducted in animal models of depression, and manipulations of the clock genes in these models have been reported to induce depression-like behavior. Strong evidence for a likely role of the clock genes in depression is found in a recent study showing that SCN-specific *Bmal1* knockdown mice exhibit depressive-like behavior [61]. However, it should be noted that SCN-specific *Bmal1* knockdown mice do not have a reduced intake in the sucrose consumption test indicative for hedonic status.

A disruption of the clock genes has a considerable effect on memory and thinking. Bearing in mind that depressed patients often suffer from cognitive deficits, Snider and colleagues demonstrated that selectively deleted *Bmal1* from excitatory forebrain neurons results in deficits in cognitive tests [62].

A differential expression of clock genes in the amygdala in the dark phase of a standard 12:12 light/dark cycle (LD) was measured in *Cry2*$^{-/-}$ mice compared to wild-type animals. Most importantly, *Cry2*$^{-/-}$ mice also exhibit anhedonic-like behavior in the sucrose preference test. In mice, a mutation in the *Per2* clock gene increased the depression- and anxiety-like behavior showed by using despair-based tests [63]. Furthermore, knockdown of the *Clock* in CA1 caused depressive-like behavior [64].

As aforementioned, the SCN is not exclusive timekeeper of the body, but rather coordinator of activity between a wide range of brain regions and peripheral sub-oscillators. Thus, the fact that depression-like behavior can be induced by manipulations with core clock genes outside the SCN raises the question about the top position of the SCN and interaction between the SCN and sub-oscillators [62].

Another approach used to investigate a role of the clock genes in the development of depression is an examination of the consequences of stress exposure on the expression of the clock genes [65–70]. All studies reported that stress significantly alters the expression pattern of the clock genes independently on applied stressors, animals strain, and time of the termination of the experiment. For instance, altered expression of the *Per2* gene in the SCN and nucleus accumbens is observed in mice exposed to chronic unpredictable mild stress [71]. In the chronic mild stress (CMS) model, *Bmal1* and *Clock* showed significantly reduced expression in the prefrontal cortex in the anhedonic-like rats [72]. Likewise, the disturbance in the circulation of corticosterone caused altered rhythm of the *Per2* gene expression in the rat brain [73, 74].

Chronological study on clock genes in rat CMS model of depression [75] demonstrated robust expression of *Per1* gene in all analyzed brain areas. The anhedonic-like behavior was associated with delayed peak in *Bmal1* expression in the SCN and completely abolished rhythmicity of the *Bmal1* expression in the nucleus accumbens. Furthermore, the expression of *Per2* was affected by CMS in all three regions of the hippocampus (DG, CA1, and CA3). In the lever, the anhedonic-like effect of CMS was pronounced in the decrease of *Per2* expression and increase in the expression of *Bmal1*. However, the rhythmicity in the expression of three clock genes was not affected by stress.

6. Stress and depression go hand in hand

6.1. When stress is assumed as a key factor in the etiology of depression

Charles B. Nemeroff said in 1996: "One way to conceptualize depression is a pathological stress response gone awry." In our days, stress is defined as any situation able to disturb physiological or psychological homeostasis [76].

However, the word stress is often incorrectly used to describe the matters of hassles in daily life. Correctly used, stress describes life experiences resulting in a specific behavior involving a serious threat to health; burnout, including anxiety and depressed mood; disturbance of sleep; difficulties handling obstacles of daily life; and abuse of stimulants and/or medicine [77]. It is important to distinguish between acute and chronic stress and between controlled and uncontrolled stress. Chronic and uncontrolled stress highly increases the risk of developing a depression.

The first response of the body to either acute or chronic stress is activation of the HPA axis [78]. A prominent feature of the HPA axis is the negative feedback mechanism upon multiple targets including the hypothalamus, the anterior pituitary, and the limbic system [79]. A substantial subgroup of depressed individuals show an increased cortisol level [80]. It has been hypothesized that dysfunction of the glucocorticoid receptors could explain the elevated cortisol level.

Glucocorticoids, the end result of stress activation of the HPA axis, are well known to affect metabolism in the liver and entrainment of the circadian rhythm in peripheral organs, including the liver, kidneys, and heart [43]. It is broadly accepted that stress activates the HPA axis and that depression is likely to be induced by stress. However, a big conundrum in the modern stress research is why some people are able to cope with a certain intensity of stress exposure and others are not.

6.2. How to successfully cope with stress

How to handle exposure to stress? The keyword is adaptation [76], and the key player is the brain determining whether a situation is threatening to the body [81]. Or as Hans Selye ("the father" of the term stress) opined: "It's not stress that kills us, it is our reaction to it."

The ability to successfully adapt to stress very much depends on early life experience. Abuse and neglect in childhood is the most prominent risk factor for ineffective stress coping [82]. A comprehensive study was done to investigate the stress-coping abilities of littermates according to the postnatal maternal care. While analyzing maternal care, the score system was used, and a score was defined by maternal behavior, where five types of maternal behaviors were distinguished: licking and/or grooming, arched-back nursing (dam shows an obvious arch in her back while nursing), blanket nursing (dam engages in nursing postures with no obvious arch in her back), passive nursing (dam is lying on her side or back while nursing her pups), and no maternal contact. Each dam received a score for a combination of leaking/grooming behavior and either one of the three nursing postures or just the nursing position alone with no leaking/grooming. The sum of 7 days of leaking/grooming scores was used as the parameter for dividing pups into groups. Dams were divided in group of low leaking/grooming mothers and in group of high leaking/grooming mothers. When pups reached age of 6 weeks, they were exposed to standard CMS procedure including initial adaptation to consume the palatable sucrose solution. It was shown that even in stress-free control conditions, offspring from damps with low maternal care activity demonstrated increased level of anxiety and rats from damps with low maternal care activity demonstrated increase in fecal concentration of corticosterone metabolites after initiation of CMS procedure. Also the susceptibility to stress was higher in animals exposed to low level of postnatal maternal care [83].

In terms of circadian rhythm and successful adaptation to the seasonal variations (mostly the related variation in daylight hours), we may assume that the coping mechanism becomes more challenged at the northern latitude of the northern hemisphere. As aforementioned, certain subtypes of depression are more pronounced at the northern latitudes, which could be the result of the challenges in the clock genes' adaptation to the seasonal variations. The sensitivity of the circadian system is also affected by daylight saving time (DST). DST is extracting one hour in spring and returns it in autumn. The major propose of this change is providing more efficient industrial usage of the sunlight. Depending on age, gender, and chronotype, the adaptation to the change in time takes from 2 to 14 days [84]. It is tempting to speculate that inaccurate correction of DST might in some rare cases result in development of depression. A study conducted in the diurnal Siberian hamster showed that shortening the length of the day induced depressive-like behavior [85].

The etiology of depression is still largely unknown although the disease has been known for centuries [86]. In recent years, evidence points to involvement of the circadian system in major depression [54].

Investigating the circadian system is of major importance in order to find new molecular targets, hence aiming for new and better treatment strategies. This does not necessarily imply novel drugs, but it could be an intervention targeting the circadian system by manipulating environmental conditions.

7. Altered 24 h rhythm in phase markers is associated with anhedonic-like behavior

Three classical phase markers (body core temperature, blood levels of melatonin, and corticosterone) exhibit a 24 h diurnal rhythm in both anhedonic-like and control rats with altered levels at specific time points of the day in the anhedonic-like rats: corticosterone levels showed an additional peak during the light (resting in nocturnal animals) phase, whereas melatonin levels were elevated during the last period of the dark phase. The core body temperature was significantly decreased during the last period of the dark phase [87].

It is reasonable to believe that the circadian machinery is involved in the depressive-like state in the CMS model, since the anhedonic-like behavior correlates well with disturbances of the circadian system, which are also observed in the clinical depression.

The most common disturbance of the circadian rhythm observed in depressed individuals is altered sleep architecture [88]. Some patients also experience a dysfunction of the HPA axis [89–91], altered 24 h rhythm of body temperature and melatonin [92], and reduced psychomotor activity [93]. These disturbances have also been reported in the CMS model of depression: sleep disturbances [94], dysfunction of the HPA axis [95], altered 24 h rhythm of core body temperature, and reduced circadian rhythm of locomotor activity [96].

However, measurements of the 24 h rhythm of phase markers are more indicative of circadian rhythm disturbances. It is important to measure the phase markers simultaneously due to their interplay and role in stress response, especially corticosterone. Furthermore, inconsistencies among the findings complicate the modeling of the chronopathology in depression [97].

The corticosterone level in animals exposed to chronic mild stress (CMS) protocol is associated with development of anhedonic-like behavior [66, 95, 98]. The additional peak in corticosterone level during the light phase has also been reported in a clinical study performed on patients with depression [99]. Landgraf and coworkers demonstrated that SCN-*Bmal1* knockdown mice after 25 h in total darkness exhibit depression-like behavior in several behavioral tests. They also have a second peak in corticosterone secretion compared to the control mice [61].

These data could provide clues to focus on another important time point for measuring the level of corticosterone/cortisol. The daily occurrence of a physiological increase in the cortisol level, associated with awakening (CAR), is normally the target point for measuring the plasma concentrations of cortisol in depressed individuals [100]. Taking into consideration the results obtained on animals, the evaluation of cortisol level at the time point, when its level is not expected to be high, might be relevant for the ongoing diagnosis of depression.

The 24 h secretion pattern of melatonin in relation to depression is mostly studied in humans, where there is a report on an elevated melatonin level in depressed individuals [31], a report on the delay in the nocturnal melatonin peak secretion in depressed patients [33], and one report on recovery of the phase shift in patient treated with melatonin [101].

Zurawek and coworkers did not find differences in levels of melatonin measured during the light phase of the light/dark cycle between resilient and anhedonic-like animals compare to the controls after 2 and 7 weeks of CMS [102]. According to the result of Christiansen et al. [87], the level of melatonin is only affected by CMS during the dark phase.

Melatonin, corticosterone/cortisol, and core body temperature are all important factors for regulating the sleep pattern. Therefore, the altered 24 h pattern in anhedonic-like rats could explain the disturbances of the sleep pattern previously demonstrated in CMS rats [94].

8. Altered expression pattern of the core clock genes might partially explain changes in the 24 h pattern of phase markers

In line with disturbances of the circadian rhythm in clinical depression, disturbances of the circadian rhythm have also been observed in animal models of depression, but only in recent years, the clock genes have been linked to the disturbances. In study of Christiansen et al. [87], expression patterns of the clock genes were significantly altered in three out of the nine brain areas investigated in the anhedonic-like rats: the hippocampus, the lateral habenula, and the nucleus accumbens. In addition, changes in clock gene expression were also observed in the liver of CMS-susceptible rats.

The diurnal pattern of *Per1* expression was significantly altered in CA1 of the hippocampus, whereas the diurnal pattern of *Per2* expression was significantly altered in all subregions of the hippocampus, in the lateral habenula, and in the liver. *Bmal1* expression was altered in the nucleus accumbens and liver [87].

At first glance, the effect of the stress paradigm on the 24 h expression pattern of the clock genes might be evaluated as minor. However, minor alterations may have a major impact. Jiang and coworkers demonstrated that specific knockdown of the clock gene called *clock* in the CA1 region of the hippocampus led to development of the depressive-like behavior. The presence of depressive-like phenotype was demonstrated by using the sucrose consumption test and the forced swim test [64]. Knockdown of *Bmal1* in the SCN also induced depressive-like behavior, such as despair and helplessness [61]. Interestingly, these SCN-specific *Bmal1*-knockdown mice did not exhibit anhedonic-like behavior tested by sucrose consumption test. Knockdown of the gene in sub-oscillators might have given rise to a different result, indicating that SCN may not be directly involved in stress-induced mood disorders, presumably due

http://dx.doi.org/10.5772/67261

to lack of the glucocorticoid receptors in the SCN [43, 103]. This might be a reason why it is widely accepted that this area of the brain is naturally protected from stress.

Remarkably, the areas of the rat brain that demonstrate most changes in the CMS paradigm are the structures, which are known to be affected in major depression.

The hippocampus is one of the most studied brain structures in depression; since the hippocampal formation is involved in learning and memory, structural and functional deficits in this area are most often accompanying clinical depression [104]. In study of Christiansen et al. [87], *Per2* was found to be most affected clock gene in the hippocampal formation. This is intriguing since Borgs and coworkers found a link between *Per2* expression and neurogenesis [105]. Using the CMS model, it has been demonstrated that anhedonic-like rats have a decreased neurogenesis [106]. The involvement of hippocampal *Per2* in the development of the depression-like state was emphasized by the results from the resilient rats showing no effect of CMS on *Per2* expression in any subregions of the hippocampus [107].

Anhedonia is a core symptom of depression, and the nucleus accumbens is a key structure in the reward circuit of the brain [108]. The observed changes in *Bmal1* expression in the nucleus accumbens could therefore be implicated in the development of the anhedonic-like behavior in the CMS model which was also underlined by the results of clock gene expression in the resilient rats where no differences were demonstrated.

The lateral habenula has been suggested to be an important structure involved in the development of the depressive phenotype [109, 110] and as a brain structure, which must be taken into consideration when studying the circadian rhythm [111]. In the CMS-exposed rats, the expression level of *Per2* in this region was altered only in anhedonic-like rats, but not in stress resilient [107]. This is indicative for the inducible character of *Per2* expression in lateral habenula and its role in the development of the depression-like phenotype.

In human postmortem brain tissue, *Bmal1* has been ranked as the gene showing the most robust circadian rhythm in control individuals. *Per2* and *Per1* were ranked on a second and a ninth place, respectively [51]. In the Li study, six regions of the human brain were investigated for diurnal expression of genes, and they reported a lack of rhythmicity in *Per1*, *Per2*, and *Bmal1* (among several other genes) in depressed individuals, indicating a disturbed circadian rhythm [51]. Although the pattern of alteration differs between studies, a link between altered clock gene expression and depression is clearly illustrated.

Thus, the inducible control for the expression of *Per2* in the hippocampus and lateral habenula as well as *Bmal1* in the nucleus accumbens and liver might be proposed to be specific for the depression-like state.

Takahashi and coworkers [112] showed that expression of *Per1* gene in the liver was highly affected by CMS after 1 week of stress exposure as demonstrated by a shifted phase in the diurnal expression, while Christiansen et al. [75] demonstrated that *Per1* was not affected by the CMS after 3.5 weeks. Together these observations indicate a highly adaptive nature of *Per1* expression, hinting that the *Per1* expression, sensitive to CMS paradigm in the beginning of the stress exposure, adapts faster than the other tested genes. Indeed, altered expression pattern of *Per2* clock gene was associated with both anhedonic-like and stress-resilient phenotypes, while changes in expression of *Bmal1* were associated with anhedonic-like phenotype only, indicating the prominent role of *Bmal1* in the development of the depressive reaction.

9. Stress resilience might be explained by the absence in disturbances in core phase markers and stress-resilient profile in the expression of clock genes

Some individuals find it challenging to live up to the conflicting roles that exist in the modern society lifestyle of today, such as performing well at home, at work, and socially. Presumably as a consequence, the number of individuals feeling burnout and depressed is increasing. However, most individuals can cope to even severe stress without getting symptoms of depression. It was shown using the CMS model of depression that part of animals exposed to chronic stress will not develop anhedonic-like behavior [113–117]. These stress-resilient animals identified by the absence of decrease in consumption of palatable sucrose solution [118] do not exhibit either loss in weight gain or cognitive deficit [119]. Neither corticosterone nor melatonin concentrations in the blood were increased as an effect of chronic (3.5 weeks) exposure to mild stressors in the stress-resilient animals, but expression of *Per2* clock gene was lower in three areas (CA1, CA3, and dentate gyrus) of the hippocampus, of the lateral habenula, and in the liver in resilient animals than unstressed controls at the late onset of the dark phase of light/dark circle [107]. Anhedonic-like animals demonstrated increased expression of *Per2* in all aforementioned brain areas, but expression level of *Per2* in the liver was also decreased [75]. It was shown that regulation of *Bmal1* expression is involved in the development of depression-like phenotype [75], but in stress-resilient rats, its expression was affected by CMS only in the nucleus accumbens [107]. Altogether, by the analysis of CMS-induced effects between stress-resilient and stress-susceptible individuals, it is possible to differentiate between general effects of stress per se and effects precipitating an anhedonic-like reaction measured on molecular, cellular, and behavioral levels. Most likely the coping mechanisms associated with stress resilience based on fast and adequate response to increased corticosterone upon the stress in turn prevent disturbances in clock gene machinery, associated with development of the depressive behavior.

10. Conclusions

Thus, the depression-like phenotype is associated with changed in 24 h rhythm of key phase markers: corticosterone, melatonin, and core body temperature. Expression of the clock genes in the master clock, the SCN, is not sensitive to stress and does not associate with the development of the depressive-like phenotype. The analysis of clock gene expression in specific brain regions and in the liver allows distinguishing between stress-resilience and stress-induced depression. The *Per1* demonstrated constitutive expression profile vigorously protected from stress effect both centrally and periphery. The analysis of *Per2* expression might be used to identify the overall effect of stress on clock gene machinery while changes in expression of *Bmal1* associated with depression-like behavior. Thereby, manipulations with circadian system might be considered as an important factor to compensate effects of chronic stress and in treatment of stress-induced pathology.

Author details

Sofie Laage Christiansen and Elena V. Bouzinova*

*Address all correspondence to: elena_bouz@hotmail.com

Translational Neuropsychiatry Unit, Department of Clinical Medicine, Health, Aarhus University, Denmark

References

[1] Lam RW. Sleep disturbances and depression: a challenge for antidepressants. Int Clin Psychopharmacol. 2006 Feb;21(Suppl 1):S25-S29.

[2] Bunney JN, Potkin SG. Circadian abnormalities, molecular clock genes and chronobiological treatments in depression. Br Med Bull. 2008;86:23-32.

[3] Katz G, Knobler HY, Laibel Z, Strauss Z, Durst R. Time zone change and major psychiatric morbidity: the results of a 6-year study in Jerusalem. Compr Psychiatry. 2002 Jan;43(1): 37-40.

[4] McClung CA. Circadian genes, rhythms and the biology of mood disorders. Pharmacol Ther. 2007 May;114(2):222-232.

[5] Lam RW, Levitt AJ, Levitan RD, Michalak EE, Cheung AH, Morehouse R, et al. Efficacy of bright light treatment, fluoxetine, and the combination in patients with nonseasonal major depressive disorder: a randomized clinical trial. JAMA Psychiat. 2016 Jan;73(1):56-63.

[6] Rusting CL, Larsen RJ. Diurnal patterns of unpleasant mood: associations with neuroticism, depression, and anxiety. J Pers. 1998 Feb;66(1):85-103.

[7] Monteleone P, Martiadis V, Maj M. Circadian rhythms and treatment implications in depression. Prog Neuropsychopharmacol Biol Psychiatry. 2011 Aug 15;35(7):1569-1574.

[8] Snyder JS, Soumier A, Brewer M, Pickel J, Cameron HA. Adult hippocampal neurogenesis buffers stress responses and depressive behaviour. Nature. 2011 Aug 3;476(7361): 458-461.

[9] Malik A, Kondratov RV, Jamasbi RJ, Geusz ME. Circadian clock genes are essential for normal adult neurogenesis, differentiation, and fate determination. PLoS One. 2015;10(10):e0139655.

[10] Valenzuela FJ, Vera J, Venegas C, Munoz S, Oyarce S, Munoz K, et al. Evidences of polymorphism associated with circadian system and risk of pathologies: a review of the literature. Int J Endocrinol. 2016;2016:2746909.

[11] Rosenthal NE, Sack DA, Gillin JC, Lewy AJ, Goodwin FK, Davenport Y, et al. Seasonal affective disorder. A description of the syndrome and preliminary findings with light therapy. Arch Gen Psychiatry. 1984 Jan;41(1):72-80.

[12] Booker JM, Hellekson CJ, Putilov AA, Danilenko KV. Seasonal depression and sleep disturbances in Alaska and Siberia: a pilot study. Arctic Med Res. 1991;Suppl:281-284.

[13] Chelminski I, Ferraro FR, Petros TV, Plaud JJ. An analysis of the "eveningness-morningness" dimension in "depressive" college students. J Affect Disord. 1999 Jan;52(1–3):19-29.

[14] Lemoine P, Guilleminault C, Alvarez E. Improvement in subjective sleep in major depressive disorder with a novel antidepressant, agomelatine: randomized, double-blind comparison with venlafaxine. J Clin Psychiatry. 2007 Nov;68(11):1723-1732.

[15] Landgraf D, McCarthy MJ, Welsh DK. Circadian clock and stress interactions in the molecular biology of psychiatric disorders. Curr Psychiatry Rep. 2014 Oct;16(10):483.

[16] Evans JA, Davidson AJ. Health consequences of circadian disruption in humans and animal models. Prog Mol Biol Transl Sci. 2013;119:283-323.

[17] San L, Arranz B. Agomelatine: a novel mechanism of antidepressant action involving the melatonergic and the serotonergic system. Eur Psychiatry. 2008 Sep;23(6):396-402.

[18] Bunney WE, Bunney BG. Molecular clock genes in man and lower animals: possible implications for circadian abnormalities in depression. Neuropsychopharmacology. 2000 Apr;22(4):335-345.

[19] Yoshii T, Vanin S, Costa R, Helfrich-Forster C. Synergic entrainment of Drosophila's circadian clock by light and temperature. J Biol Rhythms. 2009 Dec;24(6):452-464.

[20] Lucas RJ, Freedman MS, Lupi D, Munoz M, David-Gray ZK, Foster RG. Identifying the photoreceptive inputs to the mammalian circadian system using transgenic and retinally degenerate mice. Behav Brain Res. 2001 Nov 1;125(1–2):97-102.

[21] Kalsbeek A, Palm IF, La Fleur SE, Scheer FA, Perreau-Lenz S, Ruiter M, et al. SCN outputs and the hypothalamic balance of life. J Biol Rhythms. 2006 Dec;21(6):458-469.

[22] Kalsbeek A, Perreau-Lenz S, Buijs RM. A network of (autonomic) clock outputs. Chronobiol Int. 2006;23(1–2):201-215.

[23] Redman JR. Circadian entrainment and phase shifting in mammals with melatonin. J Biol Rhythms. 1997 Dec;12(6):581-587.

[24] Arendt J. Melatonin. Clin Endocrinol (Oxf). 1988 Aug;29(2):205-229.

[25] Benloucif S, Guico MJ, Reid KJ, Wolfe LF, L'hermite-Baleriaux M, Zee PC. Stability of melatonin and temperature as circadian phase markers and their relation to sleep times in humans. J Biol Rhythms. 2005 Apr;20(2):178-188.

[26] Lewy AJ, Cutler NL, Sack RL. The endogenous melatonin profile as a marker for circadian phase position. J Biol Rhythms. 1999 Jun;14(3):227-236.

[27] Lewy AJ, Sack RL. The dim light melatonin onset as a marker for circadian phase position. Chronobiol Int. 1989;6(1):93-102.

[28] Klerman EB, Gershengorn HB, Duffy JF, Kronauer RE. Comparisons of the variability of three markers of the human circadian pacemaker. J Biol Rhythms. 2002 Apr;17(2):181-193.

[29] Claustrat B, Chazot G, Brun J, Jordan D, Sassolas G. A chronobiological study of melatonin and cortisol secretion in depressed subjects: plasma melatonin, a biochemical marker in major depression. Biol Psychiatry. 1984 Aug;19(8):1215-1228.

[30] Brown R, Kocsis JH, Caroff S, Amsterdam J, Winokur A, Stokes PE, et al. Differences in nocturnal melatonin secretion between melancholic depressed patients and control subjects. Am J Psychiatry. 1985 Jul;142(7):811-816.

[31] Arendt J. Melatonin: a new probe in psychiatric investigation?. Br J Psychiatry. 1989 Nov;155:585-590.

[32] Thompson C, Franey C, Arendt J, Checkley SA. A comparison of melatonin secretion in depressed patients and normal subjects. Br J Psychiatry. 1988 Feb;152:260-265.

[33] Crasson M, Kjiri S, Colin A, Kjiri K, L'hermite-Baleriaux M, Ansseau M, et al. Serum melatonin and urinary 6-sulfatoxymelatonin in major depression. Psychoneuroendocrinology. 2004 Jan;29(1):1-12.

[34] Lewy AJ, Lefler BJ, Emens JS, Bauer VK. The circadian basis of winter depression. Proc Natl Acad Sci U S A. 2006 May 9;103(19):7414-7419.

[35] Pruessner JC, Wolf OT, Hellhammer DH, Buske-Kirschbaum A, von AK, Jobst S, et al. Free cortisol levels after awakening: a reliable biological marker for the assessment of adrenocortical activity. Life Sci. 1997;61(26):2539-2549.

[36] Streeten DH, Anderson GH, Jr., Dalakos TG, Seeley D, Mallov JS, Eusebio R, et al. Normal and abnormal function of the hypothalamic-pituitary-adrenocortical system in man. Endocr Rev. 1984;5(3):371-394.

[37] Stetler C, Miller GE. Blunted cortisol response to awakening in mild to moderate depression: regulatory influences of sleep patterns and social contacts. J Abnorm Psychol. 2005 Nov;114(4):697-705.

[38] Vreeburg SA, Hoogendijk WJ, van PJ, Derijk RH, Verhagen JC, van DR, et al. Major depressive disorder and hypothalamic-pituitary-adrenal axis activity: results from a large cohort study. Arch Gen Psychiatry. 2009 Jun;66(6):617-626.

[39] Reppert SM, Weaver DR. Molecular analysis of mammalian circadian rhythms. Annu Rev Physiol. 2001;63:647-676.

[40] Reppert SM, Weaver DR. Coordination of circadian timing in mammals. Nature. 2002 Aug 29;418(6901):935-941.

[41] Nagoshi E, Saini C, Bauer C, Laroche T, Naef F, Schibler U. Circadian gene expression in individual fibroblasts: cell-autonomous and self-sustained oscillators pass time to daughter cells. Cell. 2004 Nov 24;119(5):693-705.

[42] Abe M, Herzog ED, Yamazaki S, Straume M, Tei H, Sakaki Y, et al. Circadian rhythms in isolated brain regions. J Neurosci. 2002 Jan 1;22(1):350-356.

[43] Balsalobre A, Brown SA, Marcacci L, Tronche F, Kellendonk C, Reichardt HM, et al. Resetting of circadian time in peripheral tissues by glucocorticoid signaling. Science. 2000 Sep 29;289(5488):2344-2347.

[44] Schibler U, Ripperger J, Brown SA. Peripheral circadian oscillators in mammals: time and food. J Biol Rhythms. 2003 Jun;18(3):250-260.

[45] Durgan DJ, Hotze MA, Tomlin TM, Egbejimi O, Graveleau C, Abel ED, et al. The intrinsic circadian clock within the cardiomyocyte. Am J Physiol Heart Circ Physiol. 2005 Oct;289(4):H1530-H1541.

[46] Ramsey KM, Marcheva B, Kohsaka A, Bass J. The clockwork of metabolism. Annu Rev Nutr. 2007;27:219-240.

[47] Balsalobre A, Damiola F, Schibler U. A serum shock induces circadian gene expression in mammalian tissue culture cells. Cell. 1998 Jun 12;93(6):929-937.

[48] Mendoza J. Circadian clocks: setting time by food. J Neuroendocrinol. 2007 Feb;19(2): 127-137.

[49] Aschoff J, Fatranska M, Giedke H, Doerr P, Stamm D, Wisser H. Human circadian rhythms in continuous darkness: entrainment by social cues. Science. 1971 Jan 15;171(3967):213-215.

[50] Sequeira A, Morgan L, Walsh DM, Cartagena PM, Choudary P, Li J, et al. Gene expression changes in the prefrontal cortex, anterior cingulate cortex and nucleus accumbens of mood disorders subjects that committed suicide. PLoS One. 2012;7(4):e35367.

[51] Li JZ, Bunney BG, Meng F, Hagenauer MH, Walsh DM, Vawter MP, et al. Circadian patterns of gene expression in the human brain and disruption in major depressive disorder. Proc Natl Acad Sci U S A. 2013 Jun 11;110(24):9950-9955.

[52] Wu YH, Fischer DF, Kalsbeek A, Garidou-Boof ML, van der VJ, van HC, et al. Pineal clock gene oscillation is disturbed in Alzheimer's disease, due to functional disconnection from the "master clock". FASEB J. 2006 Sep;20(11):1874-1876.

[53] Cermakian N, Boivin DB. The regulation of central and peripheral circadian clocks in humans. Obes Rev. 2009 Nov;10Suppl 2:25-36.

[54] McClung CA. How might circadian rhythms control mood? Let me count the ways. Biol Psychiatry. 2013 Aug 15;74(4):242-249.

[55] Partonen T, Treutlein J, Alpman A, Frank J, Johansson C, Depner M, et al. Three circadian clock genes Per2, Arntl, and Npas2 contribute to winter depression. Ann Med. 2007;39(3):229-238.

[56] Kripke DF, Nievergelt CM, Joo E, Shekhtman T, Kelsoe JR. Circadian polymorphisms associated with affective disorders. J Circadian Rhythms. 2009 Jan 23;7:2.

[57] Kovanen L, Kaunisto M, Donner K, Saarikoski ST, Partonen T. CRY2 genetic variants associate with dysthymia. PLoS One. 2013;8(8):e71450.

[58] Hua P, Liu W, Chen D, Zhao Y, Chen L, Zhang N, et al. Cry1 and Tef gene polymorphisms are associated with major depressive disorder in the Chinese population. J Affect Disord. 2014 Mar;157:100-103.

[59] Shi SQ, White MJ, Borsetti HM, Pendergast JS, Hida A, Ciarleglio CM, et al. Molecular analyses of circadian gene variants reveal sex-dependent links between depression and clocks. Transl Psychiatry. 2016 Mar 1;6:e748.

[60] McCarthy MJ, Welsh DK. Cellular circadian clocks in mood disorders. J Biol Rhythms. 2012 Oct;27(5):339-352.

[61] Landgraf D, Long JE, Proulx CD, Barandas R, Malinow R, Welsh DK. Genetic disruption of circadian rhythms in the suprachiasmatic nucleus causes helplessness, behavioral despair, and anxiety-like behavior in mice. Biol Psychiatry. 2016 Dec 1;80(11):827–835

[62] Snider KH, Dziema H, Aten S, Loeser J, Norona FE, Hoyt K, et al. Modulation of learning and memory by the targeted deletion of the circadian clock gene Bmal1 in forebrain circuits. Behav Brain Res. 2016 Jul 15;308:222-235.

[63] Hampp G, Ripperger JA, Houben T, Schmutz I, Blex C, Perreau-Lenz S, et al. Regulation of monoamine oxidase A by circadian-clock components implies clock influence on mood. Curr Biol. 2008 May 6;18(9):678-683.

[64] Jiang WG, Li SX, Liu JF, Sun Y, Zhou SJ, Zhu WL, et al. Hippocampal CLOCK protein participates in the persistence of depressive-like behavior induced by chronic unpredictable stress. Psychopharmacology (Berl). 2013 May;227(1):79-92.

[65] Jiang WG, Li SX, Zhou SJ, Sun Y, Shi J, Lu L. Chronic unpredictable stress induces a reversible change of PER2 rhythm in the suprachiasmatic nucleus. Brain Res. 2011 Jul 5;1399:25-32.

[66] Blugeot A, Rivat C, Bouvier E, Molet J, Mouchard A, Zeau B, et al. Vulnerability to depression: from brain neuroplasticity to identification of biomarkers. J Neurosci. 2011 Sep 7;31(36):12889-12899.

[67] Koresh O, Kozlovsky N, Kaplan Z, Zohar J, Matar MA, Cohen H. The long-term abnormalities in circadian expression of period 1 and period 2 genes in response to stress is normalized by agomelatine administered immediately after exposure. Eur Neuropsychopharmacol. 2012 Mar;22(3):205-221.

[68] Al-Safadi S, Al-Safadi A, Branchaud M, Rutherford S, Dayanandan A, Robinson B, et al. Stress-induced changes in the expression of the clock protein PERIOD1 in the rat limbic forebrain and hypothalamus: role of stress type, time of day, and predictability. PLoS One. 2014;9(10):e111166.

[69] Erburu M, Cajaleon L, Guruceaga E, Venzala E, Munoz-Cobo I, Beltran E, et al. Chronic mild stress and imipramine treatment elicit opposite changes in behavior and in gene expression in the mouse prefrontal cortex. Pharmacol Biochem Behav. 2015 Aug;135:227-236.

[70] Schaufler J, Ronovsky M, Savalli G, Cabatic M, Sartori SB, Singewald N, et al. Fluoxetine normalizes disrupted light-induced entrainment, fragmented ultradian rhythms and altered hippocampal clock gene expression in an animal model of high trait anxiety- and depression-related behavior. Ann Med. 2016;48(1–2):17-27.

[71] Logan RW, Edgar N, Gillman AG, Hoffman D, Zhu X, McClung CA. Chronic stress induces brain region-specific alterations of molecular rhythms that correlate with depression-like behavior in mice. Biol Psychiatry. 2015 Aug 15;78(4):249-258.

[72] Calabrese F, Savino E, Papp M, Molteni R, Riva MA. Chronic mild stress-induced alterations of clock gene expression in rat prefrontal cortex: modulatory effects of prolonged lurasidone treatment. Pharmacol Res. 2016 Feb;104:140-150.

[73] Segall LA, Perrin JS, Walker CD, Stewart J, Amir S. Glucocorticoid rhythms control the rhythm of expression of the clock protein, period2, in oval nucleus of the bed nucleus of the stria terminalis and central nucleus of the amygdala in rats. Neuroscience. 2006 Jul 7;140(3):753-757.

[74] Segall LA, Amir S. Exogenous corticosterone induces the expression of the clock protein, PERIOD2, in the oval nucleus of the bed nucleus of the stria terminalis and the central nucleus of the amygdala of adrenalectomized and intact rats. J Mol Neurosci. 2010 Oct;42(2):176-182.

[75] Christiansen SL, Bouzinova EV, Fahrenkrug J, Wiborg O. Altered expression pattern of clock genes in a rat model of depression. Int J Neuropsychopharmacol. 2016 Dec 3;19(11). pii: pyw061

[76] McEwen BS. Physiology and neurobiology of stress and adaptation: central role of the brain. Physiol Rev. 2007 Jul;87(3):873-904.

[77] McEwen BS. In pursuit of resilience: stress, epigenetics, and brain plasticity. Ann N Y Acad Sci. 2016 Jun;1373(1):56-64.

[78] Checkley S. The neuroendocrinology of depression and chronic stress. Br Med Bull. 1996 Jul;52(3):597-617.

[79] De Kloet ER, Vreugdenhil E, Oitzl MS, Joels M. Brain corticosteroid receptor balance in health and disease. Endocr Rev. 1998 Jun;19(3):269-301.

[80] Pariante CM, Miller AH. Glucocorticoid receptors in major depression: relevance to pathophysiology and treatment. Biol Psychiatry. 2001 Mar 1;49(5):391-404.

[81] McEwen BS, Bowles NP, Gray JD, Hill MN, Hunter RG, Karatsoreos IN, et al. Mechanisms of stress in the brain. Nat Neurosci. 2015 Oct;18(10):1353-1363.

[82] Tost H, Champagne FA, Meyer-Lindenberg A. Environmental influence in the brain, human welfare and mental health. Nat Neurosci. 2015 Oct;18(10):1421-1431.

[83] Henningsen K, Dyrvig M, Bouzinova EV, Christiansen S, Christensen T, Andreasen JT, et al. Low maternal care exacerbates adult stress susceptibility in the chronic mild stress rat model of depression. Behav Pharmacol. 2012 Dec;23(8):735-743.

[84] Kantermann T, Juda M, Merrow M, Roenneberg T. The human circadian clock's seasonal adjustment is disrupted by daylight saving time. Curr Biol. 2007 Nov 20;17(22):1996-2000.

[85] Prendergast BJ, Nelson RJ. Affective responses to changes in day length in Siberian hamsters (*Phodopus sungorus*). Psychoneuroendocrinology. 2005 Jun;30(5):438-452.

[86] Garcia-Albea RE. Aretaeus of Cappadocia (2nd century AD) and the earliest neurological descriptions. Rev Neurol. 2009 Mar 16;48(6):322-327.

[87] Christiansen SL, Hojgaard K, Wiborg O, Bouzinova EV. Disturbed diurnal rhythm of three classical phase markers in the chronic mild stress rat model of depression. Neurosci Res. 2016 Sep;110:43-48.

[88] Perlis ML, Giles DE, Buysse DJ, Tu X, Kupfer DJ. Self-reported sleep disturbance as a prodromal symptom in recurrent depression. J Affect Disord. 1997 Feb;42(2–3):209-212.

[89] Cervantes P, Gelber S, Kin FN, Nair VN, Schwartz G. Circadian secretion of cortisol in bipolar disorder. J Psychiatry Neurosci. 2001 Nov;26(5):411-416.

[90] Srinivasan V, Smits M, Spence W, Lowe AD, Kayumov L, Pandi-Perumal SR, et al. Melatonin in mood disorders. World J Biol Psychiatry. 2006;7(3):138-151.

[91] Germain A, Kupfer DJ. Circadian rhythm disturbances in depression. Hum Psychopharmacol. 2008 Oct;23(7):571-585.

[92] Rausch JL, Johnson ME, Corley KM, Hobby HM, Shendarkar N, Fei Y, et al. Depressed patients have higher body temperature: 5-HT transporter long promoter region effects. Neuropsychobiology. 2003;47(3):120-127.

[93] Hori H, Koga N, Hidese S, Nagashima A, Kim Y, Higuchi T, et al. 24-h activity rhythm and sleep in depressed outpatients. J Psychiatr Res. 2016 Jun;77:27-34.

[94] Gronli J, Murison R, Bjorvatn B, Sorensen E, Portas CM, Ursin R. Chronic mild stress affects sucrose intake and sleep in rats. Behav Brain Res. 2004 Apr 2;150(1–2):139-147.

[95] Christiansen S, Bouzinova EV, Palme R, Wiborg O. Circadian activity of the hypothalamic-pituitary-adrenal axis is differentially affected in the rat chronic mild stress model of depression. Stress. 2012 Nov;15(6):647-657.

[96] Gorka Z, Moryl E, Papp M. Effect of chronic mild stress on circadian rhythms in the locomotor activity in rats. Pharmacol Biochem Behav. 1996 May;54(1):229-234.

[97] Olah A, Jozsa R, Csernus V, Sandor J, Muller A, Zeman M, et al. Stress, geomagnetic disturbance, infradian and circadian sampling for circulating corticosterone and models of human depression?. Neurotox Res. 2008 Apr;13(2):85-96.

[98] Taliaz D, Loya A, Gersner R, Haramati S, Chen A, Zangen A. Resilience to chronic stress is mediated by hippocampal brain-derived neurotrophic factor. J Neurosci. 2011 Mar 23;31(12):4475-4483.

[99] Bonilla-Jaime H, Retana-Marquez S, Arteaga-Silva M, Hernandez-Gonzalez M, Vazquez-Palacios G. Circadian activity of corticosterone in an animal model of depression: response to muscarinic cholinergic stimulation. Physiol Behav. 2010 Jun 16;100(4):311-315.

[100] Adam EK, Doane LD, Zinbarg RE, Mineka S, Craske MG, Griffith JW. Prospective prediction of major depressive disorder from cortisol awakening responses in adolescence. Psychoneuroendocrinology. 2010 Jul;35(6):921-931.

[101] Lewy AJ, Rough JN, Songer JB, Mishra N, Yuhas K, Emens JS. The phase shift hypothesis for the circadian component of winter depression. Dialogues Clin Neurosci. 2007;9(3):291-300.

[102] Zurawek D, Kusmider M, Faron-Gorecka A, Gruca P, Pabian P, Kolasa M, et al. Time-dependent miR-16 serum fluctuations together with reciprocal changes in the expression level of miR-16 in mesocortical circuit contribute to stress resilient phenotype in chronic mild stress—an animal model of depression. Eur Neuropsychopharmacol. 2016 Jan;26(1):23-36.

[103] Meerlo P, Sgoifo A, Turek FW. The effects of social defeat and other stressors on the expression of circadian rhythms. Stress. 2002 Feb;5(1):15-22.

[104] Videbech P, Ravnkilde B. Hippocampal volume and depression: a meta-analysis of MRI studies. Am J Psychiatry. 2004 Nov;161(11):1957-1966.

[105] Borgs L, Beukelaers P, Vandenbosch R, Nguyen L, Moonen G, Maquet P, et al. Period 2 regulates neural stem/progenitor cell proliferation in the adult hippocampus. BMC Neurosci. 2009 Mar 27;10:30.

[106] Jayatissa MN, Bisgaard C, Tingstrom A, Papp M, Wiborg O. Hippocampal cytogenesis correlates to escitalopram-mediated recovery in a chronic mild stress rat model of depression. Neuropsychopharmacology. 2006 Nov;31(11):2395-2404.

[107] Christiansen SL. Alterations of core components of the circadian system in a rat model of depression. 2016. PhD thesis. Aarhus University Press.

[108] Schlaepfer TE, Cohen MX, Frick C, Kosel M, Brodesser D, Axmacher N, et al. Deep brain stimulation to reward circuitry alleviates anhedonia in refractory major depression. Neuropsychopharmacology. 2008 Jan;33(2):368-377.

[109] Li B, Piriz J, Mirrione M, Chung C, Proulx CD, Schulz D, et al. Synaptic potentiation onto habenula neurons in the learned helplessness model of depression. Nature. 2011 Feb 24;470(7335):535-539.

[110] Cui W, Mizukami H, Yanagisawa M, Aida T, Nomura M, Isomura Y, et al. Glial dysfunction in the mouse habenula causes depressive-like behaviors and sleep disturbance. J Neurosci. 2014 Dec 3;34(49):16273-16285.

[111] Tavakoli-Nezhad M, Schwartz WJ. Hamsters running on time: is the lateral habenula a part of the clock?. Chronobiol Int. 2006;23(1–2):217-224.

[112] Takahashi K, Yamada T, Tsukita S, Kaneko K, Shirai Y, Munakata Y, et al. Chronic mild stress alters circadian expressions of molecular clock genes in the liver. Am J Physiol Endocrinol Metab. 2013 Feb 1;304(3):E301-E309.

[113] Bergstrom A, Jayatissa MN, Thykjaer T, Wiborg O. Molecular pathways associated with stress resilience and drug resistance in the chronic mild stress rat model of depression: a gene expression study. J Mol Neurosci. 2007;33(2):201-215.

[114] Bergstrom A, Jayatissa MN, Mork A, Wiborg O. Stress sensitivity and resilience in the chronic mild stress rat model of depression; an in situ hybridization study. Brain Res. 2008 Feb 27;1196:41-52.

[115] Christensen T, Bisgaard CF, Wiborg O. Biomarkers of anhedonic-like behavior, antidepressant drug refraction, and stress resilience in a rat model of depression. Neuroscience. 2011 Nov 24;196:66-79.

[116] Bouzinova EV, Moller-Nielsen N, Boedtkjer DB, Broegger T, Wiborg O, Aalkjaer C, et al. Chronic mild stress-induced depression-like symptoms in rats and abnormalities in catecholamine uptake in small arteries. Psychosom Med. 2012 Apr;74(3):278-287.

[117] Bouzinova EV, Norregaard R, Boedtkjer DM, Razgovorova IA, Moeller AM, Kudryavtseva O, et al. Association between endothelial dysfunction and depression-like symptoms in chronic mild stress model of depression. Psychosom Med. 2014 May;76(4):268-276.

[118] Wiborg O. Chronic mild stress for modeling anhedonia. Cell Tissue Res. 2013 Oct;354(1):155-169.

[119] Henningsen K, Andreasen JT, Bouzinova EV, Jayatissa MN, Jensen MS, Redrobe JP, et al. Cognitive deficits in the rat chronic mild stress model for depression: relation to anhedonic-like responses. Behav Brain Res. 2009 Mar 2;198(1):136-141.

[120] Paranjpe DA, Anitha D, Chandrashekaran MK, Joshi A, Sharma VK. Possible role of eclosion rhythm in mediating the effects of light-dark environments on pre-adult development in *Drosophila melanogaster*. BMC Dev Biol. 2005 Feb 22;5:5.

[121] Claustrat B, Brun J, Chazot G. The basic physiology and pathophysiology of melatonin. Sleep Med Rev. 2005 Feb;9(1):11-24.

[122] Cho CH. Molecular mechanism of circadian rhythmicity of seizures in temporal lobe epilepsy. Front Cell Neurosci. 2012;6:55.

Chapter 2

Brain Lateralization of Emotional Processing in Depression

Danielle M. Pereira and Azizuddin Khan

Additional information is available at the end of the chapter

http://dx.doi.org/10.5772/66828

Abstract

There are three major hypotheses regarding the lateralization of emotion in the brain—the right-hemisphere hypothesis (RHH), the valence hypothesis, and the approach-withdrawal hypothesis. The approach-withdrawal hypothesis, which is the most widely accepted, states that emotions that elicit approach behaviors are lateralized to the left hemisphere, while emotions that elicit withdrawal behaviors are lateralized to the right hemisphere. In line with this hypothesis, it has been found that persons with depression show left frontal hypoactivity and right frontal hyperactivity. This hemispheric asymmetry appears not to influence mood but rather emotional reactions to affective stimuli. That is, a person with such an asymmetry does not show a predominant negative mood, but rather heightened negative reactions to occurrences in the environment. The asymmetry may also be a biological marker of depression, with research evidence that it is found in remitted depressives and in infants of depressed mothers. Currently, research in this area focuses on identifying the mechanism underlying the link between the asymmetry and depression.

Keywords: biological marker, depression, emotion regulation, frontal hyperactivity, hemispheric asymmetry

1. Introduction

The cortex is the neuron-rich outer layer of our brains that is believed to be responsible for all higher-order mental processes. This cortex is divided anatomically into two hemispheres—left and right. While the two hemispheres are similar in appearance, they have, however, been found to show differences in function. The idea that the two hemispheres of the brain were specialized for different areas can be said to have gained popularity after Broca's discovery in the 1860s that language is lateralized to the left hemisphere. Since then, researchers have continued to explore the possibility of lateralization of other human functions. One such area of interest is human emotion. An emotion is a complex psychological state that involves three distinct components: a subjective experience, a physiological response, and a behavioral response [1]. Emotional responses, as distinguished from other responses emitted by the organism, are brief, often quick, organized, involve complex patterning across a number of different systems, and are difficult to control [2].

2. Brain lateralization of emotion: hypotheses over time

Research on brain lateralization of emotion has a long history, originating with lesion studies and more recently getting a new breath of life with the emergence of more sophisticated neuroimaging methods. In spite of research spanning over a century, strong trends in results are seen but nothing is conclusive, and debates in this area abound—this is evidence of the complicated relationship between emotions and brain and of how much scientists still have to discover about this complex organ. Views about the hemispheric specialization of emotion can now be categorized into three main hypotheses.

The oldest of these is the Right-Hemisphere Hypothesis (RHH) that, in its original version, states the right hemisphere of the brain is specialized for the perception, expression, and experience of emotion. Most work on the right-hemisphere hypothesis was done in the area of perception. For example, in lesion studies, subjects with right-hemisphere lesions were found to be more deficient than left-lesioned subjects in the perception and discrimination of emotional tones in both speech [3, 4] and emotional facial expressions [5]. With respect to the expression of emotion, several studies demonstrated that registration of emotional expression is stronger in the left than the right half of the face. Since there is contralateral control of the hemifaces, these results point to the greater role of the right hemisphere in the expression of emotion. A prolific researcher in this area was Borod, who first showed the right-hemisphere hypothesis to be superior to the handedness hypothesis that states that facial expression of emotion is dominant on the right hemiface for left-handed persons and dominant on the left hemiface for right-handed persons [6]. He later showed the right-hemisphere hypothesis to be superior to the valence hypothesis, which proposed that the dominant hemiface for emotion expression shifted as a function of valence [7]. In another study, he showed that the right-hemisphere hypothesis was upheld for facial expression irrespective of whether the expression was spontaneous or posed [8]. Later, in the history of right-hemisphere research, it has been identified that specifically posterior regions of the right-hemisphere activate during emotional perception. A study by Sato et al. [9] used Functional magnetic resonance imaging (fMRI) technique and found that the occipital and temporal cortices of the right hemisphere were activated in response to presentation of emotional faces (both happy and fearful), but not to control faces that were emotionally neutral.

However, when testing the right-hemisphere hypothesis in the area of experience, evidence has tended to be inconclusive. Most prominently, it was noticed that though studies supported right-hemisphere advantage when a negative emotion versus a control was compared, when positive emotion was studied, clear right-hemisphere dominance was not seen. Currently, therefore, when the RHH is cited, it is framed as pertaining specifically to the perception of emotion [10, 11].

An alternate hypothesis was then derived called the valence hypothesis [12]. This hypothesis holds that certain regions of the left hemisphere are specialized for the processing of positive affect, while certain regions of the right hemisphere are specialized for the processing of negative affect [2]. The bulk of evidence for the valence hypothesis came from observations in early lesion studies. It was found that persons with unilateral left hemisphere damage showed a high incidence of "catastrophic reactions," which included negative affect, tears, guilt, and pessimism about the future. At the same time, persons with unilateral right-hemisphere damage showed either indifference or euphoric reactions, characterized by inappropriate positive affect, joking and laughing, mimicry, relaxation, and a sense of well-being [13–16]. This was interpreted as evidence for contralateral inhibition, the theory that each hemisphere plays a role in inhibition of the emotional expression of the other, and when one is damaged by a lesion, the undamaged hemisphere is able to produce its emotion unchecked. The results of the lesion studies were then confirmed by studies using more precise techniques for localizing cortical lesions, such as the Wada test. In the Wada test, localized incapacitation of either hemisphere is carried out through injections of sodium-amobarbital into the left or right carotid artery. Amytal injections in the left artery produced the same catastrophic reactions, while those in the right artery produced euphoric reactions [17–21]. Moreover, Robinson et al. [22] and Starkstein et al. [23], among others, found that the closer the location of the lesion to the left frontal pole, the more severe the negative reaction observed. Thus while the posterior regions of the brain were the major focus in the right-hemisphere hypothesis studies of emotion perception, especially the temporal and occipital lobes, anterior asymmetry became the focus of studies on emotion expression and the valence hypothesis.

Attempts were made to formulate alternate explanations for the results of these studies. Gainotti [15] proposed that patients' psychological response to their own illness may account for some of the emotional asymmetries observed. Since right-hemisphere damaged patients are often unaware of their deficits, a condition called anosognosia, perhaps they do not show negative reactions to their own illness like left-hemisphere-lesion patients do. However, this hypothesis does not account for the WADA test results. Since the right- versus left-hemisphere incapacitation in those studies is merely temporary, the negative emotions observed in left-hemisphere injection patients is not a reaction to an illness. Other researchers theorized that the emotional asymmetry observed in these studies should be interpreted as symptoms of emotional communication disorder rather than differences in emotional experience. Since emotional prosody or speech and emotions in facial expressions are right-hemisphere lateralized, right-hemisphere damaged patients cannot show depressive reactions and may be seen as indifferent. However, a study by Gasparrini et al. [24] refuted this hypothesis. The Minnesota Multiphasic Inventory (MMPI) was administered to both left- and right-hemisphere damaged patients. It was found that left-hemisphere-damaged patients scored significantly higher on the depression scale than right-hemisphere-damaged patients. Since the MMI does not require emotionally intoned speech or facial expressions, the observed difference in scale scores can be assumed to reflect difference in emotional experience.

With the emergence of electroencephalography (EEG) as a research technique, a large amount of supportive evidence was obtained for the valence hypothesis. In this method, brain waves are recorded by amplifying voltage differences between electrodes placed on the scalp. There are four major types of brain waves that are identified—alpha, beta, gamma, and theta. Alpha waves are associated with relaxation, cortical idling, and cognitive inactivity. Thus power in the alpha-band frequency is considered a reverse measure of tonal brain activation, that is, if greater frequency of alpha waves is recorded in a particular brain area, activity of that area is assumed to be low. Davidson et al. [25] published the first paper linking positive and negative affect to frontal EEG asymmetry, where relative left frontal activity was associated with positive affect, while relative right frontal activity was associated with negative affect. This was followed by a large number of EEG studies yielding results that supported the association between the frontal left hemisphere and positive emotion and frontal right hemisphere and negative emotion. For example, Tomarken et al. [26] recorded EEG data from normal participants and administered the Positive and Negative Affect Schedule (PANAS) to them. Results showed that subjects who were characterized by relatively greater left versus right frontal activation reported increased positive and decreased negative affect. The reverse was found in subjects with the opposite pattern of asymmetry. Versions of the valence hypothesis now differ as to whether the right-left distinction is seen for all emotional processing or whether perception of emotion irrespective of valence is right-hemisphere dominant.

One limitation of the valence hypothesis, however, is its inability to account for the lateralization of anger, which though popularly considered a negative emotion has found to be left-hemisphere dominant [27]. This limitation is dealt with in the third and most recent hypothesis regarding the lateralization of emotion, namely the approach-withdrawal hypothesis. The approach-withdrawal hypothesis is phylogenetically relevant because it looks at emotion from the point of view of the evolutionary purpose it serves. In terms of motivation, emotions serve one of two purposes—to elicit approach behaviors or withdrawal behaviors in response to stimuli or situations. For example, happiness and anger elicit approach behaviors, to celebrate or to attack, respectively. Both fear and disgust elicit withdrawal behaviors—fear elicits the flight response, while disgust elicits a termination response, the shutting down of input from a sense organ. This hypothesis states that the left and right anterior regions of the left and right hemispheres are dominant for approach and withdrawal behaviors, respectively. The left frontal cortex is important for intention, planning, and regulation, which are important components of approach behaviors. The right prefrontal cortex has links to behavioral inhibition, which is important for withdrawal. According to Davidson [28], there are individual differences in approach versus withdrawal temperament, which are state-like and stable over time, and these can be linked to stable differences in baseline measures of activation asymmetry in the anterior regions of the brain. Approach versus withdrawal behavior to specific stimuli is then superimposed on this state. Since positive emotion motivates approach behavior and negative emotion is associated with withdrawal, this hypothesis overlaps significantly with the valence hypothesis. However, the approach-withdrawal hypothesis overcomes one of the limitations of the valence hypothesis in that it accounts for left-hemisphere dominance of the emotion anger, which elicits approach behavior even though it is considered to have negative valence. However, one limitation of the approach-withdrawal hypothesis is the contradiction of associating the right hemisphere with withdrawal behavior when it has been established that the right hemisphere is responsible for creativity, which is definitely an approach behavior [29].

3. Depression and hemispheric asymmetry

If the approach-withdrawal theory of emotion lateralization is accepted, with its view that the frontal right hemisphere is specialized for withdrawal emotions and the frontal left hemisphere for approach emotions, one could then reasonably hypothesize that clinical depression would show a stronger relationship with the frontal right hemisphere than the frontal left hemisphere. This hypothesis has been supported by a variety of studies using the different techniques for exploring brain lateralization.

Early studies of patients with unilateral lesions who developed clinical depression analyzed the location of lesion in relationship to the severity of the depression experienced. Two features of the lesions were repeatedly associated with greater likelihood for depression—first, that it was located in the left rather than the right hemisphere and second, that it was located in anterior rather than posterior regions [30–33]. Interpreting this in the light of contralateral inhibition it appears that when the inhibitory capacity of the frontal left hemisphere is affected due to damage, the right hemisphere is free to produce negative emotion unchecked. The results of these and other similar studies led Ross and Rush [34] to theorize that depression may be initiated by structures in the right hemisphere.

While lesion studies were informative, it was necessary to determine whether the hypothesized relationship between depression and the right hemisphere could be demonstrated in patients with intact brain function. With the development of more advanced methods, studies using the technique of positron emission tomography (PET) found relatively greater right frontal than left frontal activation in depressed subjects [35, 36]. But the largest body of evidence in favor of this relationship comes from studies using the electroencephalography method to study the brains of persons with depression. Early studies by Tucker et al. [37] and Schaffer et al. [38] found a relationship between relatively greater right frontal activation and higher scores on self-report measures of depression among students. Henriques and Davidson [39] found that clinically depressed patients had relatively greater right-hemisphere activation than left-hemisphere activation, which was not seen in controls. The same asymmetry has been observed in multiple studies of persons with depression [40–44].

Moreover, it appears that this demonstrable anterior hemispheric asymmetry could function as a trait marker for depression. There are two main lines of evidence supporting this claim. First, studies that have compared EEG activation in currently depressed patients to remitted patients have found no significant difference in the asymmetry seen in the two groups [39, 43, 45, 46]. Thus, right-hemisphere hyperactivation is not only limited to depressed patients with currently active symptoms, suggesting a trait-like rather than state-like nature. Allen et al. [46] examined resting EEG alpha in 30 women diagnosed in major depression at four-week intervals over a course of 8–16 weeks. They found lesser left than right-hemisphere activity (characterized by greater left than right alpha-band activity) in these women, and this asymmetry showed over the course of the study, evidence that this is a fairly stable characteristic of depression.

Second, developmental research studies have found that the anterior asymmetry can be seen in infants as well. In a study by Davidson and Fox [47], EEG recordings from 10-month-old infants showed that there is relatively greater right frontal activation in infants who cry in response to maternal separation as compared to those who do not cry. Studies have found that 1-month-old infants [48] and 3-month-old infants [49] of depressed mothers with anterior asymmetry also have relatively greater right-hemisphere activation than left-hemisphere activation. Moreover, this asymmetry is stable across time. A second study by Jones et al. [50] found that right-hemisphere hyperactivation in 3-month-old infants of depressed mothers persisted when the infants were tested at age 3 years. Thus evidence appears to support the idea that right-hemisphere activation is a biological vulnerability marker for depression that is inherited. One should note though, that twin studies [51, 52] have found that only 11–28% of the variance of frontal alpha power asymmetry in children and 27% of variance in adults is accounted for by genetics.

However, there are some inconsistencies in results across studies, suggesting that the lateralization of emotion suggested by the approach-withdrawal hypothesis and the relationship between anterior hemispheric asymmetry and depression are not as simple as they seem. Gainotti [53] reviewed a number of studies on left- versus right-brain-damaged patients that did not find a clear difference in lateralization of emotion. Similarly, several groups have failed to demonstrate lateralization of emotion and anterior asymmetry in depression in EEG studies [54, 55]. A meta-analysis by Wager et al. [56] found limited support for a simple valence-based lateralization of emotion in the brain and concluded that lateralization of emotion in the brain is more complex and region-specific than early theories proposed.

Davidson [28] argued that the reason for differing results in some studies is that anterior cerebral asymmetry predisposes positive versus negative responses only in the presence of a specific emotion elicitor. Thus studies using the same procedure may yield different results because the participants' emotional behavior depends not merely on asymmetry in frontal cortical activation but more importantly on the emotion elicitors present during the experiment, which differ from study to study. Davidson and Fox [47] demonstrated that in healthy controls, baseline anterior asymmetry in the hemispheres predicts emotional reactions to a specific emotional challenge but is unrelated to general emotional state. In a study by Tomarken et al. [57], baseline EEG was recorded, following which participants were made to view film clips designed to elicit either positive or negative emotion. They found that baseline frontal right-hemisphere activation was associated with a heightened negative affective reaction to the negative film clips. Similarly, Wheeler et al. [58] measured baseline EEG recordings of participants at two separate occasions three weeks apart. Following the second recording, participants were shown brief positive and negative emotional film clips. Researchers found that if a recorded frontal asymmetry was stable across the three-week interval, then those participants with greater left frontal activation reported more intense positive affect in response to the positive film clips, while those participants with greater right frontal activation reported more intense negative affect in response to the negative film clips. In other words, these studies demonstrate that anterior hemispheric asymmetry predisposes affective reactions in the individual and not mood. Thus, the right-hemisphere hyperactivity seen in depression would not precipitate a negative mood, but would be associated with heightened negative affective reactions to stimuli.

Recent research in the area has focused on determining what underlies the link between this particular hemispheric asymmetry and depression. The above distinction between mood and emotional reaction makes it tenable that the frontal right and left hemispheres are involved in emotion regulation. That is, the anterior asymmetry observed in depression may not be associated with differences in production of negative emotions, but may be associated with a difficulty regulating negative affective reactions to stimuli. Pereira and Khan [59] tested this hypothesis using a tachistoscopic task that measured the ability to disengage attention from affective stimuli. In this experiment, emotion regulation was not defined as a higher-order strategy like cognitive restructuring. Rather, the focus was on the basic cognitive process of attention, specifically the ability to disengage or inhibit attention to a stimulus. This ability can be considered highly relevant in the context of emotion regulation since an important first step in regulating emotion is shifting attention away from the emotion-producing stimulus. Furthermore, impaired disengagement of attention is a repeatedly found cognitive deficit in depression. In the experimental task used in this study, affective stimuli (pictures in one version of the task and words in another version) were primed to either the left or right hemisphere by manipulating position of presentation on the screen. This was followed by immediate presentation of the affective primed stimulus with a neutral stimulus both in the center of the screen, one below the other. In half the trials, the neutral stimulus was placed over the affective stimulus, in the other half, the affective stimulus was placed over the neutral one. Participants had to indicate the position of the neutral stimulus by pressing either the "Up" or "Down" arrow keys, thus requiring them to shift attention away from the primed affective one. Apart from the visual field presentation, valence of the affective stimulus was manipulated at two levels—positive and negative. The dependent variable measured was the reaction time of the participants in pressing the key on each trial. The assumption was that the longer the reaction time, the longer the time taken by the participant to disengage from the affective stimulus and note the location of the neutral stimulus. The same task was given to both clinically depressed participants and healthy controls to perform. In controls, a distinct right-hemisphere advantage was seen for disengaging attention, that is, shorter reaction times for affective stimuli primed to the left visual field irrespective of valence. This was found to be in line with research that has identified right-hemisphere structures as the seat of behavioral inhibition. In the depressed group, however, this right-hemisphere advantage was not observed. These results support the inference that the right-hemisphere hyperactivity seen in depression is due to some dysfunction of the inhibition system.

Author details

Danielle M. Pereira and Azizuddin Khan*

*Address all correspondence to: khanaziz@iitb.ac.in

Psychophysiology Laboratory, Department of Humanities and Social Sciences, Indian Institute of Technology Bombay, Mumbai, Maharashtra, India

References

[1] Hockenbury, D. H., & Hockenbury, S. E. (2007). Discovering psychology. New York: Worth Publishers.

[2] Davidson, R. J. (1984). Affect, cognition, and hemispheric specialization. In Izard, C. E., Kagan, J., & Zajonc, R. (Eds.), Emotions, cognition, and behavior (pp. 320–365). New York: Cambridge University Press.

[3] Heilman, K., Scholes, R., & Watson, R. (1975). Auditory affective agnosia: Disturbed comprehension of affective speech. Journal of Neurology, Neurosurgery, and Psychiatry, 38, 69–72.

[4] Tucker, D. M., Watson, R. T., & Heilman, K. M. (1977). Discrimination and evocation of affectively intoned speech in patients with right parietal disease. Neurology, 27, 947–950.

[5] DeKosky, S., Heilman, K. M., Bowers, D., & Valenstein, E. (1980). Recognition and discrimination of emotional faces and pictures. Brain and Language, 9, 206–214.

[6] Borod, J. C., & Caron, H. S. (1980). Facedness and emotion related to lateral dominance, sex, and expression type. Neuropsychologia, 18, 237–241.

[7] Borod, J., Kent, J., Koff, E., & Martin, C., et al. (1988). Facial asymmetry while posing positive and negative emotions: Support for the right hemisphere hypothesis. Neuropsychologia, 26, 759–764.

[8] Borod, J. C., Koff, E., & White, B. (1983). Facial asymmetry in posed and spontaneous expressions of emotion. Brain and Cognition, 2, 165–175.

[9] Sato, W., Kochiyama, T., & Yoshikawa, S. (2004). Enhanced neural activity in response to dynamic facial expressions of emotion: An fMRI study, *Cognitive Brain Research*, 20, 81–91.

[10] Smith, S. D., & Bulman-fleming, M. B. (2005). An examination of the right-hemisphere hypothesis of the lateralization of emotion. Brain and Cognition, 57, 210–213.

[11] Killgore, W. D. S., & Yurgelun-Todd, D. A. (2007). The right-hemisphere and valence hypotheses: Could they both be right (and sometimes left)?. Social Cognitive and Affective Neuroscience, 2(3), 240–250.

[12] Silberman, E. K., & Weingartner, H. (1986). Hemispheric lateralization of functions related to emotion. Brain and Cognition, 5, 322–353.

[13] Alford, L. B. (1933). Localization of consciousness and emotion. American Journal of Psychiatry, 89(4), 789–799.

[14] Goldstein, K. (1939). The organism: An holistic approach to biology, derived from pathological data in man. New York: American Book.

[15] Gainotti, G. (1972). Emotional behavior and hemispheric side of the lesion. Cortex, 8, 41–55.

[16] Sackheim, H., Decina, P., & Malitz, S. (1982). Functional brain asymmetry and affective disorders. Adolescent Psychiatry, 10, 320–335.

[17] Terzian, H. (1964). Behavioral and EEG effects of intracarotid sodium amytal injections. Acta Neurochirurgica, 12, 230–240.

[18] Alema, G., Rosadini, G., & Rossi, G. F. (1961). Psychic reactions associated with intracarotid Amytal injection and relation to brain damage. Excerpta Medica, 37, 154–155.

[19] Perria, P., Rosadini, G., & Rossi, G. F. (1961). Determination of side of cerebral dominance with Amobarbital. Archives of Neurology, 4, 175–181.

[20] Rossi, G. F., & Rosadini, G. R. (1967). Experimental analyses of cerebral dominance in man. In Millikan, D. H., & Darley, F. L. (Eds.), Brain mechanisms underlying speech and language. New York: Grune & Stratton.

[21] Lee, G. P., Loring, D. W., Meader, K. J., & Brooks, B. B. (1990). Hemispheric specialization for emotional expression : A reexamination of results from intracarotid administration of sodium amobarbital. Brain and Cognition, 12, 267–280.

[22] Robinson, R. G., Kubos, K. L., Starr, L. B., Reo, K., & Price, T. R. (1984). Mood disorders in stroke patients. Importance of location of lesion. Brain, 107, 81–93.

[23] Starkstein, S. E., Robinson, R. G., & Price, T. R. (1987). Comparison of cortical and subcortical lesions in the production of poststroke mood disorders. Brain, 110, 1045–1059.

[24] Gasparrini, W. G., Satz, P., Heilman, K., & Coolidge, F. L. (1978). Hemispheric asymmetries of affective processing as determined by the Minnesota Multiphasic Personality Inventory. Journal of Neurology, Neurosurgery and Psychiatry, 41, 470–473.

[25] Davidson, R. J., Schwartz, G. E., Saron, C., Bennett, J., & Goleman, D. J. (1979). Frontal versus parietal EEG asymmetry during positive and negative affect. Psychophysiology, 16, 202–203.

[26] Tomarken, A. J., Davidson, R. J., Wheeler, R. W., & Doss, R. (1992). Individual differences in anterior brain asymmetry and fundamental dimensions of emotion. Journal of Personality and Social Psychology, 62, 676–687.

[27] Harmon-Jones, E., & Allen, J. J. (1998). Anger and frontal brain activity: EEG asymmetry consistent with approach motivation despite negative affective valence. Journal of Personality and Social Psychology, 74(5), 1310–1316.

[28] Davidson, R. J. (1992). Anterior cerebral asymmetry and the nature of emotion. Brain and Cognition, 20, 125–151.

[29] Rotenberg, V. S. (2004). The peculiarity of the right-hemisphere function in depression : Solving the paradoxes. Progress in Neuro-Psychopharmacology & Biological Psychiatry, 28, 1–13.

[30] Benson, D. F. (1973). Psychiatric aspects of aphasia. British Journal of Psychiatry, 123, 555–566.

[31] Benson, D. (1979). 1. Aphasia, alexia and agraphia. New York: Churchill-Livingstone.

[32] Robinson, R. G., & Benson, D. F. (1981). Depression in aphasic patients: Frequency, severity and clinical-pathological correlations. Brain and Language, 14, 282–291.

[33] Robinson, R. G., & Szetela, B. (1981). Mood change following left hemispheric brain injury. Annals of Neurology, 9, 447–453.

[34] Ross, E. D., & Rush, A. (1981). Diagnosis and neuroanatomical correlates of depression in brain-damaged patients: Implications for a neurology of depression. Archives of General Psychiatry, 38, 1344–1354.

[35] Bench, C. F., Friston, K. J., Brown, R. G., Scott, L. C., Frackowiak, R. S. J., & Dolan, R. J. (1993). Regional cerebral blood flow in depression measured by positron emission tomography: The relationship with clinical dimensions. Psychological Medicine, 23, 579–590.

[36] Martinot, J. L., Hardy, P., Feline, A., Huret, J., Mazoyer, B., Attar-Levy, D., Pappata, S., & Syrota, A. (1990). Left prefrontal glucose hypometabolism in the depressed state: A confirmation. American Journal of Psychiatry, 147, 1313–1317.

[37] Tucker, D. M., Stenslie, C. E., Roth, R. S., & Shearer, S. L. (1981). Right frontal lobe activation and right hemisphere performance. Archives of General Psychiatry, 38, 169–174.

[38] Schaffer, C. E., Davidson, R. J., & Saron, C. (1983). Frontal and parietal electroencephalogram asymmetry in depressed and nondepressed subjects. Biological Psychiatry, 18, 753–762.

[39] Henriques, J. B., & Davidson, R. J. (1991). Left frontal hypoactivity in depression. Journal of Abnormal Psychology, 100, 535–545.

[40] Allen, J. J., Iacono, W. G., Depue, R. A., & Arbisi, P. (1993). Regional electroencephalographic asymmetries in bipolar seasonal affective disorder before and after exposure to bright light. Biological Psychiatry, 33, 642–646.

[41] Bruder, G. E., Stewart, J. W., Mcgrath, P. J., Deliyannides, D., & Quitkin, F. M. (2004). Dichotic listening tests of functional brain asymmetry predict response to fluoxetine in depressed women and men. Neuropsychopharmacology, 29, 1752–1761.

[42] Debener, S., Beauducel, A., Nessler, D., Brocke, B., Heilemann, H., & Kayser, J. (2000). Is resting anterior EEG alpha asymmetry a trait marker for depression?. Neuropsychobiology, 41(1), 31–37.

[43] Gotlib, I. H., Ranganath, C., & Rosenfeld, J. P. (1998). Frontal EEG alpha asymmetry, depression, and cognitive functioning. Cognition & Emotion, 12(3), 449–478.

[44] Vuga, M., Fox, N. A., Cohn, J. F., George, C. J., Levenstein, R. M., & Kovacs, M. (2006). Long-term stability of frontal electroencephalographic asymmetry in adults with a history of depression and controls. International Journal of Psychophysiology, 59(2), 107–115.

[45] Henriques, J. B., & Davidson, R. J. (1990). Regional brain electrical asymmetries discriminate between previously depressed and healthy control subjects. Journal of Abnormal Psychology, 99, 22–31.

[46] Allen, J. J. B., Urry, H. L., Hitt, S. K., & Coan, J. A. (2004). The stability of resting frontal electroencephalographic asymmetry in depression. Psychophysiology, 41(2), 269–280.

[47] Davidson, R. J., & Fox, N. A. (1989). Frontal brain asymmetry predicts infants' response to maternal separation. Journal of Abnormal Psychology, 98, 127–131.

[48] Jones, N. A., Field, T., Fox, N. A., Lundy, B., & Davalos, M. (1997). EEG activation in 1-month-old infants of depressed mothers. Development and Psychopathology, 9(3), 491–505.

[49] Field, T., Fox, N. A., Pickens, J., & Nawrocki, T. (1995). Relative right frontal EEG activation in 3 to 6 month old infants of "depressed" mothers. Developmental Psychology, 31, 358–363.

[50] Jones, N. A., Field, T., Davalos, M., & Pickens, J. (1997). EEG stability in infants/children of depressed mothers. Child Psychiatry and Human Development, 28(2), 59–70.

[51] Anokhin, A. P., Heath, A. C., & Myers, E. (2006). Genetic and environmental influences on frontal EEG asymmetry: A twin study. Biological Psychology, 71, 289–295

[52] Gao, Y., Tuvblad, C., Raine, A., Lozano, D. I., & Baker, L. A. (2009). Genetic and environmental influences on frontal EEG asymmetry and alpha power in 9–10-year-old twins. Psychophysiology, 46(4), 787–796.

[53] Gainotti, G. (1989). Disorders of emotions and affect in patients with unilateral brain damage. In Boiler, E., & Grafman, J. (Eds.), Handbook of neuropsychology (Vol. 3, pp. 345–361). Amsterdam: Elsevier.

[54] Collet, L., & Duclaux, R. (1987). Hemispheric lateralization of emotions: Absence of electrophysiological arguments. Physiology and Behavior, 40, 215–220.

[55] Reid, S. A., Duke, L. M., & Allen, J. J. B. (1998). Resting frontal electroencephalographic asymmetry in depression : Inconsistencies suggest the need to identify mediating factors. Psychophysiology, 35, 389–404.

[56] Wager, T. D., Phan, K. L., Liberzon, I., & Taylor, S. F. (2003). Valence, gender, and lateralization of functional brain anatomy in emotion: A meta-analysis of findings from neuroimaging. Neuroimage, 19, 513–531.

[57] Tomarken, A. J., Davidson, R. J., & Henriques, J. B. (1990). Resting frontal brain asymmetry predicts affective responses to films. Journal of Personality and Social Psychology, 59(4), 791–801.

[58] Wheeler, R. E., Davidson, R. J., & Tomaken, A. J. (1993). Frontal brain asymmetry and emotional reactivity: A biological substrate of affective style. Psychophysiology, 30, 82–89.

[59] Pereira, D. M., & Khan, A. (2015). Hemispheric specialization of impaired disengagement of attention in depression: A tachistoscopic method. Laterality: Asymmetries of Body, Brain and Cognition, DOI: 10.1080/1357650X.2015.1090444.

Section 2

Depression and Comorbidity

Chapter 3

Anxiety and Depression in Cardiovascular Surgery

Yuko Okamoto and Noboru Motomura

Additional information is available at the end of the chapter

http://dx.doi.org/10.5772/67064

Abstract

Although anxiety and depression are psychological risk factors for coronary artery disease (CAD), psychological aspect in patients with cardiovascular surgery has been less considered. Cognitive and psychological deficit has been still concerning in spite of notable improvement of cardiovascular surgery using cardiopulmonary bypass perfusion. The purpose of this chapter review is to discuss recent data concerning the prevalence and trend of anxiety and depression of patients with cardiovascular surgery and to introduce the nonpharmacological intervention studies. The prevalence of anxiety and depression of patients after cardiovascular surgeries has varied from 10 to 60% and has been likely higher than that of general people. From the limited studies about patients over 6 months after surgery, we guessed the followings about the trends of anxiety and depression of patients with CABG without any other additional intervention programs before/after surgery: (1) patients improved scores of anxiety and depression 3–6 months after surgery, (2) anxiety decreased considerably for about 6 months after CABG and then leveled out for some time, (3) depression remained a bit higher 6 months and more after CABG. Patients' longitudinal psychological conditions would have been influenced by not only invasive cardiovascular surgery but also life events. The nonpharmacology intervention would have improved patients' psychological conditions. Further research is needed to clarify the long-term psychological outcome and to develop the effective intervention programs toward patients with cardiovascular surgery.

Keywords: cardiovascular, surgery, depression, anxiety

1. Introduction

Although Rozanski et al. extensively reviewed and found that anxiety and depression were psychological risk factors for coronary artery disease (CAD), and that depression was particularly a predictor of cardiac events, many research studies have been focused on psychological outcomes of patients with heart failure, myocardial infraction, and acute coronary syndromes among CAD [1]. Results of cardiovascular surgery have improved remarkably in recent years but psychological aspect in patients who underwent cardiovascular surgery has been less considered.

The advances in both surgical and cardiopulmonary bypass perfusion techniques regarding cardiovascular surgery have been reducing mortality and relieving from patients' symptoms. However, cognitive and psychological deficit has been concerning [2–4]. Selnes and Gottesman suggested that late cognitive changes do occur and these changes are not specific to coronary artery bypass grafting surgery (CABG) or more specifically to the use of cardiopulmonary bypass [2].

Therefore, out of various kinds of cardiovascular surgery using cardiopulmonary bypass, we found out coronary artery bypass grafting surgery (CABG), valve surgery (VS), ventricular device surgery (VDS), and thoracic aortic surgery (TAS) in terms of the adults' main cardiovascular surgery and then reviewed the psychological outcomes of patients with these four surgical procedures. The articles in English language journals were collected by using PubMed (accessed on August 26, 2016) with keywords as follows: CABG, VS, TAS, VDS, cardiovascular surgery, depression, and anxiety. We also described nonpharmacological intervention research.

2. Anxiety and depression in coronary artery bypass grafting surgery (CABG)

Coronary artery bypass grafting (CABG) surgery is performed more frequently than other cardiovascular surgeries. Tully and Baker reviewed about depression, anxiety, and cardiac morbidity outcomes after coronary artery bypass surgery [5]. They suggested the followings: (1) the approximate percentage of coronary artery bypass graft (CABG) surgery patients affected by depression (i.e., major, minor, dysthymia) was between 30 and 40% immediately leading up to and after surgery, (2) both depression and anxiety raised the risk for mortality and morbidity after CABG surgery independent of medical factors, although the behavioral and biological mechanisms are poorly understood, and (3) although neither depression nor anxiety seem to obviously affect neuropsychological dysfunction, depression contributes to a risk for incident delirium.

Compared to psychological condition immediately leading up to and after CABG surgery, the midterm or long-term psychological condition in CABG patients was limited. The long-term psychological research in CABG patients using a hospital anxiety and depression scale (HADS) has only been performed by Ben-Noun [6], who reported HADS results in 132 CABG patients in Israel 7–22 years after surgery. He found the following: (1) anxiety: 31 (23.5%) patients were severe, and two (1.5%) were mild, and (2) depression: 25 (18.9%) patients were severe and three (2.3%) were mild. We examined the psychological outcome of patients at intervals of 1–5 years after CABG using HADS and found that six (8.7%) of them were mild anxiety and five (7.2%) were severe anxiety [7]. Regarding to depression, seven (10.1%) were mild and seven (10.1%) were severe. Compared with his findings, our figures for patients in the significant range (HAD-A>10) of both anxiety and depression were lower, while our figures for patients in the borderline range (7<HAD-A<11) were higher. Ben-Noun's study was conducted in Israel and there are long-running conflicts between the Palestinian and the Israeli people. Mataria et al. have found that the chronic and entrenched conflict over generations has resulted in a lower QOL for the population living in the occupied Palestinian territory [8]. Although it might be simplistic to suggest that these factors could influence levels of anxiety and depression, we thought that they might have been a contributing influence to the psychological aspects of the subjects of Ben-Noun's study.

Table 1 presents the trends of HADS anxiety and depression in studies preCABG to post-CABG [4, 9–12]. Some studies have found that CABG patients without any intervention programs after surgery had improved scores of both anxiety and depression 3–6 months after CABG [4, 10, 11]. The means for anxiety 3–6 months after surgery in these studies ranged from 4.2 to 4.9, similar to our results, and for depression from 2.6 to 4.25. Our interpretation of these findings was that anxiety would decrease considerably for about 6 months after CABG and then level out for some time. In contrast, values for depression in our study ranged on the high side. That might have been influenced somewhat by life events because most patients were elderly and had survived several years after their operation [13].

In our study, the prevalence of anxiety and depression in patients more than 1 year after CABG was similar to other reported studies. The exceptions were Ben-Noun's study [6] in Israel with the added effect of war-like conditions. Although most of the previous research on psychological aspects in CABG patients examined them within 1 year of the operation, in which case proximity to the surgical event might have had a great influence, our findings help to understand midterm psychological transitions, and suggest the possible need for further research such as a longitudinal study carried out over several years to better quantify the process of psychological transition.

3. Anxiety and depression in valve surgery (VS)

Not only CABG but valve surgery (VS) procedures also are more common surgical treatment for cardiovascular disease, and some patients need both procedures. There were less psychological studies of patients with VS than those of patients with CABG.

The postoperative psychological research studies revealed that some of patients with VS and/or CABG had anxiety and depression, which had associated with their self-management performance, readmission. Williams et al found that about 30% of patients before CABG and/or VS had moderate to high levels of anxiety [14]. Fredericks et al. reviewed systematically about psychological condition of patients with CABG and/or VS and revealed that moderate to severe levels of anxiety and depression existed during the first month of home recovery and appeared to have an effect on their performance of selfmanagement behaviors [15]. Sibilitz et al. conveyed a nationwide cohort study on patients 1 year after valve surgery in Denmark and found that anxiety and depression were present in 13.6 and 13.8%, respectively (hospital anxiety and depression scale score ≥8) and that higher HADS-D scores was one of

References/nation	No. of subject	Anxiety and depression score: means (standard deviations)					Results
		Before surgery/ treatment	1–2 months after surgery/treatment	3–6 months after surgery/treatment	7–11 months after surgery/treatment	1 year or more after surgery/ treatment	
Cross-sectional study							
Okamoto et al. [7]/Japan	49 pts: TAS 79 pts: CABG Anxiety & depression: HADS					1–5 years TA CABG A: 4.0(3.1) 4.7(4.2) D: 5.5(3.7) 5.0(4.5)	
Oterhals et al. [17]/Denmark	593 pts: AVR 369 pts: AVR+CABG Anxiety & depression: HADS					1–13 years AVR AVR+CABG A: 3.78(3.58) 3.57(3.69) D: 3.67(3.39) 4.33(3.53)	
Longitudinal study							
Thornton et al. [4]/UK	71 male pts; CABG Anxiety & depression: HADS	1 week before surgery A: 6.4 D: 4.7	2 months A: 5.3 D: 3.4	6 months A: 4.9 D: 2.6			Anxiety and depression decreased
Hallas et al. [9]/UK	22 pts: CABG Anxiety & depression: HADS	1 week before surgery A: 8.4(4.6) D: 5.7(2.9)	2 months A: 3.4(2.3) D: 2.0(2.2)				Anxiety and depression decreased
Höfer et al. [10]/Austria	432 pts: CAD (CMT: 96 pts, PCI: 60 pts, CABG: 121pts) Anxiety & depression: HADS	Before angiography/ treatment CABG CMT PCI A: 6.40(3.42) 6.52(3.62) 6.55(3.67) D: 4.61(3.14) 4.88(3.38) 5.06(3.86)	1 month CABG CMT PCI A: 5.04(3.97) 6.04(4.12) 5.61(3.25) D: 4.26(3.34) 5.27(4.25) 4.27(3.52)	3 months CABG CMT PCI A: 4.25(3.67) 6.55(4.42) 5.90(3.85) D: 4.25(3.80) 5.30(4.37) 4.59(3.98)			Anxiety and depression in CABG decreased

http://dx.doi.org/10.5772/67064

References/nation	No. of subject	Anxiety and depression score: means (standard deviations)					Results
		Before surgery/ treatment	1–2 months after surgery/treatment	3–6 months after surgery/treatment	7–11 months after surgery/treatment	1 year or more after surgery/ treatment	
Amonn et al. [25]/Swiitzerland	51 pts: transcatheter aortic valve implantation (TAVI) 93 pts: surgical aortic valve replacement (AVR) Anxiety & depression: HADS					A mean follow-up of 15 + 10 months <u>TAVI AVR</u> A: 4.0(4) 4.0(3) D: 4.7(4) 4.0(4)	
Brouwers et al. [32]/Netherlands	54 pts: LVAD Anxiety: Generalized Anxiety Disorder, GAD-7 (range: 0–21, cutoff: 10/9) Depression: Patient Health Questionnaires, PHQ-9 (range: 0–27, cutoff;10/9)		3–4 weeks A: 4.4(4.8) D: 6.9(4.5)	3 and 6 months: data was not shown		12 months: data was not shown	Higher scores on anxiety and depression over time were associated with poor health status
Reynard et al. [29]/ USA	66 pts: LVAD Anxiety: Generalized Anxiety Disorder, GAD-7 (range: 0–21, cutoff: 10/9) Depression: Patient Health questionnaire, PHQ-9 (range: 0–27, cutoff;10/9)	Before implantation A: 10.4(6.2) D: 12.1(7.5)	Follow-up (median:54 days, mean:126 days) A: 3.4(4.3) D: 5.7(5.4)				Anxiety and depression scores improved after LVAD implantation and remained stable up to 1 year

References/nation	No. of subject	Anxiety and depression score: means (standard deviations)					Results
		Before surgery/ treatment	1–2 months after surgery/treatment	3–6 months after surgery/treatment	7–11 months after surgery/treatment	1 year or more after surgery/ treatment	
Randomized controlled trial							
Furze et al.[42]/UK	I. 100 pts: first elective CABG C: 104 pts: first elective CABG Intervention: cognitive-behavioral intervention, nurse counseling Anxiety: the State Trait Anxiety Inventory, STAI (range: 20–80, cutoff: 55/54) Depression: cardiac depression scale, CDS (range: 26–182, cutoff: 95 or 100)	Baseline: placed on the elective waiting list I C A: 40.01(12.30) 41.52(12.69) D: 93.09(22.12) 96.78(23.49) 8 weeks after baseline I C A: no data D: 81.96 93.37					Anxiety and depression in the intervention group decreased
Rollman et al. [43]/ USA	I_1: 150 depressed postCABG, telephone-delivered collaborative care I_2: 151 depressed post-CABG, usual care C: 151 nondepressed post-CABG, usual care Depression: the 17-items Hamilton Rating scale for depression (range: 0–68, cutoff: 8/7)		Discharge I_1 I_2 C D: 16.5(7.1) 15.9(6.9) 3.1(2.6)		8 months I_1 I_2 C D: 9.0(0.7) 11.4(0.7) no data		Anxiety and depression in the I_1 group decreased compared to the I_2 group
Lie et al. [11]/ Norway	185 pts: elective CABG Intervention: a structured informational and psychological support by a skilled nurse at each patient's home Anxiety & depression: HADS	I C A: 5.7(3.8) 6.5(4.1) D: 3.8(3.6) 4.5(3.7)	6 weeks I C A:3.2(3.2) 3.9(3.6) D:3.2(2.8) 3.6(3.6)	6 months I C A:3.1(3.6) 4.2(4.2) D:2.7(3.1) 3.5(4.0)			Anxiety and depression in both group decreased. Not significant differences in two groups

http://dx.doi.org/10.5772/67064

References/nation	No. of subject	Anxiety and depression score: means (standard deviations)					Results
		Before surgery/ treatment	1–2 months after surgery/treatment	3–6 months after surgery/treatment	7–11 months after surgery/treatment	1 year or more after surgery/ treatment	
Trzcieniecka-Green et al. [12]/UK	50 pts: MI 50 pts: CABG Intervention: therapist-guided relaxation and stress management Anxiety & depression: HADS		2–3 months (Baseline) I C A: 7.50(3.3) 7.38(4.0) D: 4.32(2.5) 4.70(3.6)	5–6 months (3 months) I C A: 5.94(3.3) 7.60(4.2) D: 3.36(3.0) 4.68(3.7)	8–9 months (6 months) I C A: 5.73(3.1) no data D: 2.98(2.4) no data		Anxiety and depression in the intervention group decreased
Nonrandomized controlled trial							
Kugler et al. [36]/ Germany	I: 34 LVAD C: 36 LVAD Intervention: nutrition management, physical recondition program, psychosocial support and counseling Anxiety & depression: HADS		6 weeks I C A:2.0(0.6) 5.0(0.6) D:4.5(0.6) 4.0(0.5)	6 months: shown in only graph		12 and 18 months: shown in only graph	Anxiety level in the control group increased over time relative to the intervention group. No significant changes and differences in depression level were detected for both groups.

A: HADS anxiety; D: HADS depression; I: intervention group, C:control; TAS: thoracic aortic surgery, CABG: coronary artery bypass grafting, CMT: continuous medical treatment, PCI: percutaneous coronary intervention group.

Table 1. The level of anxiety and depression before/after surgery.

the associated factors to readmission [16]. Oterhals et al. examined mid-term/long-term self-reported health status of patients 1 year or more after aortic valve replacement and/or CABG. The mean assessment interval since surgery was 6 years (range: 1–13 years) [17]. Compared to patients 1–5 years after CABG or TAS, the averages of both anxiety and depression were low (**Table 1**). That might be because the interval period after surgery in Oterhals's study was much longer and psychological conditions of dead patients after surgery were unknown, who was afraid of moderate/severe level of anxiety/depression.

There were a few prospective studies to patients with VS and/or CABG. Preoperative anxiety and/or depression would predict postoperative patient's QOL [18–20], persistent depression [21], worse physical condition [18], mortality, and mobidity [14]. These studies did not show the mean of anxiety and depression of patients with VS and/or CABG.

Since transcatheter valve implantation (TVI) was carried out for the first time in 2002 [22], its technology has been developing speedily. TVI is less-invasive treatment than valve surgery and more patients with a high-risk for valve surgery have been undergoing TVI. Psychological research about patients who underwent TVI also has begun recently. Elmalem et al. found that 37% of patients had improved anxiety and depression both 1 month and 6 months after TVI [23]. Two studies reported that anxiety/depression had become better after TVI but there were no differences about anxiety/depression between TVI and valve surgery patients after adjustment for baseline characteristics [24, 25]. Amonn et al. assessed anxiety and depression using HADS after a mean follow-up of 15 + 10 months and found that anxiety disorder was present in 5.7% of AVR and 12.9% of TAVI patients and that depression disorder was apparent in 17.1% of AVR and 12.9% of TAVI patients [25].

4. Anxiety and depression in ventricular device surgery (VDS)

Left ventricular assist devices (LVADs) have been developing dramatically, and patient with end-stage heart failure can be treated it as a destination therapy or as a bridge to transplant. Continuous-flow LVADs have reduced incidence of morbidity and mortality [26]. The number of psychological research has been increasing gradually.

Brouwers et al. reviewed systematically 16 quantitative studies with a sample size ≥10 that examined the impact of LVAD therapy, including both pulsatile devices and continuous-flow devices, on patients' health status and anxiety/depression [27]. They suggested that patients had improved their health status, anxiety, and depression in the first few months after LVAD implantation and that those scores of patients receiving LVAD therapy were still below for physical, social, and emotional functioning compared with transplant recipients. After Brouwer's study, some studies [28, 29] found decreasing of anxiety/depression after introducing LVADs, but two studies [30, 31], whose sample size were about 10, did not found the significant improvement in anxiety and depression. Higher scores on anxiety/depression over time were associated with poor health status [32] and rehospitalization [33]. Family of patients with LVAD was also increasing anxiety or depression level after implantation [34, 35].

Nonrandomized intervention research was carried out by Kugler et al. [36]. It used behavior-modifying strategies and consisted of nutrition management by a dietician, physical reconditioning program, psychosocial support, and counseling. Thirty-four patients were intervention group and 36 patients were the control group. Baseline was 6 weeks after implantation and patients were reassessed at 6, 12, and 18 months during their LVAD support time. The anxiety level in the control group increased over time relative to the intervention group. No significant changes and differences in depression level were detected. Physical health status scores in the intervention group increased significantly but mental health status scores in both groups did not change.

Patients' psychological status would improve after LVAD implantation. That might be because they relieve from bad physical conditions. Heart failure patients are not always in good physical conditions and have psychological problems. After implantation, patients need anticoagulation treatment and monitoring function of devices, etc., in addition to maintain healthier lifestyle for secondary prevention. Moreover, they have several risk-like malfunction device, infection, neurological dysfunction ,etc. So patients need both physical and psychological care, and further research needs to develop better programs for their support.

5. Anxiety and depression in thoracic aortic surgery (TAS)

Instead of recent improvement of the surgical treatment of cardiovascular diseases, the hospital mortality rate for thoracic aortic surgery (TAS) is still high (approximately 10.5% in Japan) compared to coronary artery bypass grafting (CABG) surgery (approximately 2.2% in Japan) [37]. Some adverse complications of TAS can be extremely serious (e.g., brain injury, spinal cord injury, and bleeding, etc.). TAS is included in the same surgical repertoire as CABG in terms of open heart surgery, but it has a worse postoperative outcome. A few studies on psychological outcome have been conducted in TAS patients [38].

We surveyed 190 patients who underwent TAS or CABG at intervals of 1–5 years after the procedure, and then analyzed 128 patients with TAS (n = 49) or CABG (n = 79) as the primary surgery. Psychological outcomes were assessed using the hospital anxiety and depression scale (HADS). The incidence of mild (8–10) anxiety in TAS and CABG patients was five (11.6) vs. six (8.7%), respectively, and depression was present in nine (19.1%) and seven (10.1%), respectively. The incidence of severe (11 and more over) anxiety in TAS and CABG patients was four (8.5) vs. seven (10.1%), respectively, and depression was present in four (8.5%) and seven (10.1%), respectively. Psychological outcomes scores for the two groups did not differ significantly [7].

Fukuhara and Suzuki has reported that 5.6% of general Japanese (n = 2279) were suffering from severe depression using HADS on nationwide survey [39]. Kawakami reviewed that the prevalence of major depression among community-dwelling Japanese was 1–2% and estimated that of those who were seen in a general practice in Japan were approximately 5% [40]. He also reviewed that the prevalence of major depression among community-dwellers in the world was 1–8%. Compared to these community-based previous studies, not only CABG patients, as we mentioned in Section 2, but also TAS patients at intervals of 1–5 years after the procedure might have higher percentage of depressive patients. Psychological outcomes in TAS patients might improve in the same manner as CABG.

Emergency surgery was revealed only one significant factor associated with depression in TAS, and there was no significant associated factor about anxiety in TAS. Symptoms such as chest pain and fatigue were associated with both anxiety and depression in CABG. We found that the frequency in TAS survivors was nearly equal to that in CABG survivors and that variables related to anxiety or depression were not so apparent in TAS patients compared to CABG patients [7]. Interestingly, emergency operation was related to depression in TAS patients but not in CABG patients, suggesting that awareness of their disease before surgery was related to depression. Generally speaking, many patients with TAS are asymptomatic until diagnosis [41], and some of them had to undergo an emergency operation just after diagnosis. This might have had an influence on depression in TAS patients who had undergone an emergency operation even if they had survived for some time afterward. On the other hand, even if CABG patients had undergone an emergency operation, they were already aware of their own disease because of the presence of symptoms such as chest pain, and shortness-of-breath. This would have lessened the impact on their psychological wellbeing after surgery compared with the TAS patients.

Interestingly, there were no variables on symptoms significantly related to anxiety and depression in TAS patients but there were some significantly related to both anxiety and depression in CABG patients. As Herrmann has suggested in cardiac patients HADS anxiety or depression is correlated with some symptoms, but there have been differences across studies [13]. Although the reason why TAS patients with some symptoms were not positive for anxiety or depression remains unknown, we suggest that TAS patients might be less fearful of death postoperatively because the surgical removal or repair of their aortic lesion had, in their minds, reduced the risk of a cardiac event, even if they were still experiencing some symptoms.

6. Nonpharmacological intervention

Several behavioral and psychological RCT intervention research have been carried out toward patients with CABG. In this section, one research prior to CABG surgery and three ones after CABG surgery were introduced.

Regarding intervention before CABG surgery, Furze et al. evaluated the addition of a brief, cognitive-behavioral RCT intervention (the HeartOp Program) to routine nurse counseling for people waiting for CABG surgery [42]. When patients in the intervention group were introduced, for the first time, in the outpatient clinic by nurses using a booklet that covered cardiac myths and misconceptions, reducing risk factors for secondary prevention and recovery process after surgery. The HeartOp program also included relaxation program on audiotape or CD and a diary for recording activity and risk factor reduction goals. Nurses followed by telephone at 1, 3, and 6 weeks and then monthly until they were hospitalized. At

8 weeks after baseline, there were no differences in anxiety. There were significant differences in depression (cardiac depression scale: difference = 7.79, $p = 0.008$, 95% CI = 2.04–13.54). There was no data after CABG surgery.

Rollman et al. had tested the effectiveness of an 8 month, biweekly, nurse-led telephone-delivered collaborative care for post-CABG depression vs. usual physician care in a randomized controlled trial [43]. A nurse telephoned to intervention patients and provided basic psycho-education about depression and its impact on cardiac disease using a workbook. The nurse also adjusted antidepressant drugs prescribed under their physicians' direction, monitoring, and referral to a mental health specialist if needed. Not only physical functioning (duke activity status index: delta=4.6 points, 95% CI=1.9-7.3) but also depression (Hamilton rating scale for depression: delta=3.1 points; 95% CI=1.3-4.9) had improved at 8 months after baseline. But the average HRQL and physical functioning of intervention patients did not recover that of the nondepressed comparison group.

Lie et al. evaluated the effects of a home-based intervention program (HBIP) on anxiety and depression 6 months after CABG [11]. An HBIP for the intervention group was performed 2 and 4 weeks after surgery. A skilled nurse provided education about angina symptoms, medication, how to emergency attention, and so on with emotional support at 2 and 4 weeks after surgery. Although the improvements of anxiety and depression symptoms did not differ significantly between the groups, on 6-week and 6-month follow-ups, significant improvements in anxiety and depression symptoms were found in both groups.

Trzcieniecka-Green and Steptoe assessed the impact of group-based stress management training on emotional wellbeing, functional status, social activity, and chest pain in patients following acute myocardial infarction or coronary bypass surgery, within a randomized controlled trial [12]. Experimental patients underwent a 10 group-based weekly sessions about relaxation-based stress management program by therapists. Significantly greater improvements in both anxiety and depression were found in the experimental groups than control groups, and improvements were maintained at 6-month follow-up.

In the nonpharmacology intervention, patients received behavioral and psychological education, etc., by a nurse or a therapist, and their depression would be improved after the intervention. Further research needed to clarify the effect of intervention group compared to control group.

7. Conclusion and implication for future research

The prevalence of anxiety and depression of patients after cardiovascular surgeries has varied from 10 to 60% and has been likely higher than that of general people. Although there were several studies about patients within 6 months after surgery, studies about patients over 6 months after surgery were limited. From the limited studies about patients over 6 months after surgery, we guessed the followings about the trends of anxiety and depression of patients with CABG without any other additional intervention programs before/after surgery: (1) patients improved scores of anxiety and depression 3–6 months after surgery,

(2) anxiety decreased considerably for about 6 months after CABG and then leveled out for some time, and (3) depression remained a bit higher 6 months and more after CABG. Patients' longitudinal psychological conditions would have been influenced by not only invasive cardiovascular surgery using cardiopulmonary bypass perfusion techniques but also life events. The nonpharmacology intervention consisting of behavioral and psychological education, etc., by a nurse or a therapist would have improved patients' psychological conditions. Further research needed to clarify the long-term psychological outcome and to develop the more effective intervention programs toward patients with cardiovascular surgery.

Author details

Yuko Okamoto[1] and Noboru Motomura[2*]

*Address all correspondence to: noboru@motomura.org

1 Japanese Red Cross College of Nursing, Shibuya-ku, Tokyo, Japan

2 Toho University Medical Center, Sakura Hospital, Sakura-City, Chiba, JAPAN

References

[1] Rozanski A, Blumenthal JA, Kalpan J. Impact of psychological factors on the pathogenesis of cardiovascular disease and implications for therapy. Circulation 1999;99:2192–2217.

[2] Selnes OA, Gottesman RF. Neuropsychological outcomes after coronary artery bypass grafting. J Int Neuropsychol Soc. 2010 Mar;16(2):221–6. DOI: 10.1017/S1355617709991196. Epub 2009 Dec 11.

[3] Miyairi T, Takamoto S, Kotsuka Y, Takeuchi A, Yamanaka K, Sato H. Neurocognitive outcome after retrograde cerebral perfusion. Ann Thorac Surg. 2004 May;77(5):1630–3. DOI: 10.1016/j.athoracsur.2003.10.007

[4] Thornton EW, Groom C, Fabri BM, Fox MA, Hallas C, Jackson M. Quality of life outcomes after coronary artery bypass graft surgery: relationship to neuropsychologic deficit. J Thorac Cardiovasc Surg. 2005 Oct;130(4):1022–7.

[5] Tully PJ, Baker RA. Depression, anxiety, and cardiac morbidity outcomes after coronary artery bypass surgery: a contemporary and practical review. J Geriatr Cardiol. 2012 Jun;9(2):197–208. DOI: 10.3724/SP.J.1263.2011.12221.

[6] Ben-Noun LL. Coronary artery bypass grafting: long-term psychological and social outcomes. J Anxiety Disord 1999;13:505–512.

[7] Okamoto Y, Motomura N, Murashima S, Takamoto S. Anxiety and depression after thoracic aortic surgery or coronary artery bypass. Asian Cardiovasc Thorac Ann. 2013 Feb;21(1):22–30. DOI: 10.1177/0218492312444283.

[8] Mataria A, Giacaman R, Stefanini A, Naidoo N, Kowal P, Chatterji S. The quality of life of Palestinians living in chronic conflict: assessment and determinants. Eur J Health Econ 2009;10(1):93–101.

[9] Hallas CN, Thornton EW, Fabri BM, Fox MA, Jackson M. Predicting blood pressure reactivity and heart rate variability from mood state following coronary artery bypass surgery. Int J Psychophysiol 2003;47:43–55.

[10] Höfer S, Doering S, Rumpold G, Oldridge N, Benzer W. Determinants of health-related quality of life in patients with coronary artery disease. Eur J Cardiovasc Prev Rehabil 2006;13:398–406.

[11] Lie I, Arnesen H, Sandvik L, Hamilton G, Bunch EH. Effects of a home-based intervention program on anxiety and depression 6 months after coronary artery bypass grafting: a randomized controlled trial. J Psychosom Res 2007;62(4):411–18. DOI: 10.1016/j.jpsychores.2006.11.010

[12] Trzcieniecka-Green A, Steptoe A. The effects of stress management on the quality of life of patients following acute myocardial infarction or coronary bypass surgery. Eur Heart J 1996;17:1663–1670.

[13] Herrmann C. International experiences with the hospital anxiety and depression scale—a review of validation data and clinical results. J Psychosom Res 1997;42(1):17–44.

[14] Williams JB, Alexander KP, Morin JF, Langlois Y, Noiseux N, Perrault LP, Smolderen K, Arnold SV, Eisenberg MJ, Pilote L, Monette J, Bergman H, Smith PK, Afilalo J. Preoperative anxiety as a predictor of mortality and major morbidity in patients aged >70 years undergoing cardiac surgery. Am J Cardiol. 2013 Jan 1;111(1):137-42. doi: 10.1016/j.amjcard.2012.08.060.

[15] Fredericks S, Lapum J, Lo J. Anxiety, depression, and self-management: a systematic review. Clin Nurs Res. 2012 Nov;21(4):411–30. DOI: 10.1177/1054773812436681. Epub 2012 Apr 3. Review. PubMed PMID: 22473273.

[16] Sibilitz KL, Berg SK, Thygesen LC, Hansen TB, Køber L, Hassager C, Zwisler AD. High readmission rate after heart valve surgery: a nationwide cohort study. Int J Cardiol. 2015;189:96–104. DOI: 10.1016/j.ijcard.2015.04.078. Epub 2015 Apr 11.

[17] Oterhals K, Hanssen TA, Haaverstad R, Nordrehaug JE, Eide GE, Norekvål TM. Factors associated with poor self-reported health status after aortic valve replacement with or without concomitant bypass surgery. Eur J Cardiothorac Surg. 2015 Aug;48(2):283–92. DOI: 10.1093/ejcts/ezu425. Epub 2014 Nov 19.

[18] Kohlmann S, Rimington H, Weinman J. Profiling illness perceptions to identify patients at-risk for decline in health status after heart valve replacement. J Psychosom Res. 2012 Jun;72(6):427–33. DOI: 10.1016/j.jpsychores.2012.03.002. Epub 2012 Apr 2.

[19] Markou AL, de Jager MJ, Noyez L. The impact of coronary artery disease on the quality of life of patients undergoing aortic valve replacement. Interact Cardiovasc Thorac Surg. 2011 Aug;13(2):128–32. DOI: 10.1510/icvts.2011.269209. Epub 2011 May 17.

[20] Rimington H, Weinman J, Chambers JB. Predicting outcome after valve replacement. Heart. 2010 Jan;96(2):118–23. DOI: 10.1136/hrt.2008.160010. Epub 2009 Jun 4.

[21] Patron E, Messerotti Benvenuti S, Palomba D. Preoperative and perioperative predictors of reactive and persistent depression after cardiac surgery: a three-month follow-up study. Psychosomatics. 2014 May-Jun;55(3):261–71. DOI: 10.1016/j.psym.2013.12.011. Epub 2013 Dec 23.

[22] Cribier A, Eltchaninoff H, Bash A, Borenstein N, Tron C, Bauer F, Derumeaux G, Anselme F, Laborde F, Leon MB. Percutaneous transcatheter implantation of an aortic valve prosthesis for calcific aortic stenosis: first human case description. Circulation. 2002 Dec 10;106(24):3006–8. PMID: 12473543

[23] Elmalem S, Dumonteil N, Marcheix B, Toulza O, Vellas B, Carrie D, Nourhashemi F. Health-related quality of life after transcatheter aortic valve implantation in elderly patients with severe aortic stenosis. J Am Med Dir Assoc. 2014 Mar;15(3):201–6. DOI: 10.1016/j.jamda.2013.11.010. Epub 2014 Jan 18.

[24] Völler H, Salzwedel A, Nitardy A, Buhlert H, Treszl A, Wegscheider K. Effect of cardiac rehabilitation on functional and emotional status in patients after transcatheter aortic-valve implantation. Eur J Prev Cardiol. 2015 May;22(5):568–74. DOI: 10.1177/2047487314526072. Epub 2014 Feb 27.

[25] Amonn K, Stortecky S, Brinks H, Gahl B, Windecker S, Wenaweser P, Carrel T, Huber C. Quality of life in high-risk patients: comparison of transcatheter aortic valve implantation with surgical aortic valve replacement. Eur J Cardiothorac Surg. 2013 Jan;43(1):34–41; discussion 41–2. DOI: 10.1093/ejcts/ezs173. Epub 2012 Apr 24.

[26] Kugler C, Malehsa D, Tegtbur U, Guetzlaff E, Meyer AL, Bara C, Haverich A, Strueber M. Health-related quality of life and exercise tolerance in recipients of heart transplants and left ventricular assist devices: a prospective, comparative study. J Heart Lung Transplant. 2011 Feb;30(2):204–10. DOI: 10.1016/j.healun.2010.08.030. Epub 2010 Oct 27.

[27] Brouwers C, Denollet J, de Jonge N, Caliskan K, Kealy J, Pedersen SS. Patient-reported outcomes in left ventricular assist device therapy: a systematic review and recommendations for clinical research and practice. Circ Heart Fail. 2011 Nov;4(6):714–23. DOI: 10.1161/CIRCHEARTFAILURE.111.962472. Epub 2011 Sep 9. Review.

[28] Estep JD, Starling RC, Horstmanshof DA, Milano CA, Selzman CH, Shah KB, Loebe M, Moazami N, Long JW, Stehlik J, Kasirajan V, Haas DC, O'Connell JB, Boyle AJ,Farrar DJ, Rogers JG; ROADMAP Study Investigators. Risk assessment and comparative effectiveness of left ventricular assist device and medical management in ambulatory

heart failure patients: results from the roadmap study. J Am Coll Cardiol. 2015 Oct 20;66(16):1747–61. DOI: 10.1016/j.jacc.2015.07.075.

[29] Reynard AK, Butler RS, McKee MG, Starling RC, Gorodeski EZ. Frequency of depression and anxiety before and after insertion of a continuous flow left-ventricular assist device. Am J Cardiol. 2014 Aug 1;114(3):433–40. DOI: 10.1016/j.amjcard.2014.05.015. Epub 2014 May 17.

[30] Mapelli D, Cavazzana A, Cavalli C, Bottio T, Tarzia V, Gerosa G, Volpe BR. Clinical psychological and neuropsychological issues with left ventricular assist devices (LVADs). Ann Cardiothorac Surg. 2014 Sep;3(5):480–9. DOI: 10.3978/j.issn.2225-319X.2014.08.14.

[31] Casida JM, Parker J. A preliminary investigation of symptom pattern and prevalence before and up to 6 months after implantation of a left ventricular assist device. J Artif Organs. 2012 Jun;15(2):211–4. DOI: 10.1007/s10047-011-0622-4. Epub 2011 Nov 26.

[32] Brouwers C, de Jonge N, Caliskan K, Manintveld O, Young QR, Kaan A, Kealy J, Denollet J, Pedersen SS. Predictors of changes in health status between and within patients 12 months post left ventricular assist device implantation. Eur J Heart Fail. 2014 May;16(5):566–73. DOI: 10.1002/ejhf.75. Epub 2014 Mar 11.

[33] Snipelisky D, Stulak JM, Schettle SD, Sharma S, Kushwaha SS, Dunlay SM. Psychosocial characteristics and outcomes in patients with left ventricular assist device implanted as destination therapy. Am Heart J. 2015 Nov;170(5):887–94. DOI: 10.1016/j.ahj.2015.08.012. Epub 2015 Aug 16. PubMed PMID: 26542496;

[34] Brouwers C, Caliskan K, de Jonge N, Theuns DA, Constantinescu A, Young QR, Cannon C, Denollet J, Pedersen SS. A comparison of the health status and psychological distress of partners of patients with a left ventricular assist device versus an implantable cardioverter defibrillator: a preliminary study. Heart Lung. 2015 Jan-Feb;44(1):27–32. DOI: 10.1016/j.hrtlng.2014.10.007. Epub 2014 Nov 20.

[35] Brouwers C, Denollet J, Caliskan K, de Jonge N, Constantinescu A, Young Q, Kaan A, Pedersen SS. Psychological distress in patients with a left ventricular assist device and their partners: an exploratory study. Eur J Cardiovasc Nurs. 2015 Feb;14(1):53–62. DOI: 10.1177/1474515113517607. Epub 2013 Dec 17.

[36] Kugler C, Malehsa D, Schrader E, Tegtbur U, Guetzlaff E, Haverich A, Strueber M. A multi-modal intervention in management of left ventricular assist device outpatients: dietary counselling, controlled exercise and psychosocial support. Eur J Cardiothorac Surg. 2012 Dec;42(6):1026–32. DOI: 10.1093/ejcts/ezs206. Epub 2012 Jun 21.

[37] Sakata R, Fujii Y, Kuwano H. Thoracic and cardiovascular surgery in Japan during 2008: annual report by the Japanese association for thoracic surgery. Gen Thorac Cardiovasc Surg 2010;58:356–383.

[38] Olsson C, Thelin S. Quality of life in survivors of thoracic aortic surgery. Ann Thorac Surg 1999;67:1262-67.

[39] Fukuhara S., Suzuki Y. Manual pf SF-36v2 Japanese version: iHope International Inc. Kyoto, 2004, 2015. P138.

[40] Kawakami N. Major depression in Japan and the world: state-of-art in epidemiology. In [Igaku no Ayumi: Bessatu Saisin Utsubyo no Subete] (Japanese). 2010;3:42–46.

[41] Kouchoukos NT, Blackstone EH, Doty DB. Diseases of the thoracic arteries and veins. In Kirklin JW, Barratt-Boyes. Cardiac Surgery: Morphology, Diagnostic Criteria, Natural History, Techniques, Results, and Indications. 3rd edition. New York, Churchill Livingstone, 2003, vol. 2, pp. 1824–1857.

[42] Furze G, Dumville JC, Miles JN, Irvine K, Thompson DR, Lewin RJ. "Prehabilitation" prior to CABG surgery improves physical functioning and depression. Int J Cardiol. 2009 Feb 6;132(1):51–8. DOI: 10.1016/j.ijcard.2008.06.001. Epub 2008 Aug 15.

[43] Rollman BL, Belnap BH, LeMenager MS, Mazumdar S, Houck PR, Counihan PJ, Kapoor WN, Schulberg HC, Reynolds CF 3rd. Telephone-delivered collaborative care for treating post-CABG depression: a randomized controlled trial. JAMA. 2009 Nov 18;302(19):2095–103. DOI: 10.1001/jama.2009.1670. Epub 2009 Nov 16.

Chapter 4

Chronic Pain and Depression

Aleksandra A. Karapetyan and
Hovhannes M. Manvelyan

Additional information is available at the end of the chapter

http://dx.doi.org/10.5772/66671

Abstract

Today, it is clear that chronic pain and depression are closely related. Depression can cause pain, and chronic pain can cause depression too. According to the American Pain Foundation, about 32 million people in the U.S. report have had pain lasting longer than 1 year. Statistical international data prove that more than half of the patients with pain are depressed or have mood swings, and on average, 65% of depressed people also complain of pain. Patients simultaneously suffering of chronic pain and limited independence are especially vulnerable. Fibromyalgia (FM) is one of the most common chronic pain syndromes, affecting 15 up to 5% of world population, is characterized as diffuse widespread body pain, with definite tender points and clinical features, and also triggers the development of depression. Depression severity in patients with FM worsens severity of pain. Depressive disorders are observed in approximately 90% of patients with FM. Pain triggers development of depressive conditions in patients with chronic character of pain, and time course of disease shows certain pattern of increasing of severity of depression and worsens long term outcomes. Patients with chronic pain must be evaluated for depression, and successful management of pain must include treatment of depressive mood too.

Keywords: chronic pain, fibromyalgia, chronic fatigue syndrome, depression and depressive symptoms

1. Introduction

The results of medical investigations conducted in the field of pain unveiled the unbearable burden of living with chronic or long-term pain. Moreover, simultaneous suffering of pain and depression makes that burden heavier and worsens prognosis. Patients with depression emotionally suffer from more severe pain, and in the case of primary pain, they more prone to develop depression.

It is widely accepted that chronic pain is often defined as any pain lasting more than 12 weeks. Whereas acute pain is a normal sensation that alerts about possible injury or inflammation, chronic pain is very different. Chronic pain persists often for several months or even longer.

Chronic pain may arise from an initial injury of the tissue, or there may be an ongoing cause, such as illness. However, there may also be no clear cause. Other health problems, such as fatigue, sleep disturbance, decreased appetite, and mood changes, often accompany chronic pain. Chronic pain may limit patient's motility, which can reduce flexibility, strength, and stamina. This difficulty in carrying out important and enjoyable activities can lead to some level of disability and despair.

Chronic pain can prevent sleep and cause patients to awaken frequently at night. This lack of sleep further results in daytime fatigue and low productivity. The ongoing pain will cause additional irritation and make it difficult to deal with others.

Depression is one of the most common psychological issues people facing who suffer from chronic pain, and it often complicates the patient's conditions and treatment. Current statistical data prove that according to the American Pain Foundation, about 32 million people in the U.S. report have had pain lasting longer than 1 year; from one-quarter to more than half of the population that complain of pain to their doctors are depressed, and on average, 65% of depressed people also complain of pain.

People whose pain limits their independence are especially likely to become depressed.

Because depression in patients with chronic pain frequently goes undiagnosed, it often goes untreated. Pain symptoms and complaints take center stage on most doctor visits; bad mood is usually ignored or explained as the result of long-lasting pain, but not simultaneously growing medical condition. The result is depression along with sleep disturbances, loss of appetite, lack of energy, and decreased physical activity, which may make pain much worse.

Fibromyalgia (FM) is a chronic pain syndrome characterized by generalized pain, the presence of specific tender points (small areas of excessive pain, localized in different areas of the body), sleep disorders, and severe chronic fatigue. In the general population of patients with chronic widespread pain, FM occupies an exclusive position that affects between 2 and 5% of the general population in the United States and is diagnosed more often in women (7:1) [1–4].

A significant increase in the number of patients with a variety of persistent pain syndromes and certain advances in the diagnosis and management of FM expressed interest in the problem of pain by the medical community; the nature of the priority of this syndrome raises the FM up to the level of medical and social problems. Latter is confirmed by a number of international and national associations of fibromyalgia and pain research.

Considering that the known clinical symptoms become apparent, the FM complex problem is more complex than just muscle pain. Persistence of sets of clinical symptoms, not based on morphological, biochemical, and other changes, allows considering FM as somatoform disorder. In addition, there is strong evidence of lowering the threshold of pain sensitivity in

http://dx.doi.org/10.5772/66671

patients with FM. At the same time, clinical application of different methods, such as neurosensory potential testing, revealed that the mechanical allodynia in patients with FM is not restricted to tender points and is prevalent [5].

Currently, an increase in the number of FM investigators is considered as functional and somatic pathology [6, 7].

It becomes obvious that the FM is a more complex problem than just widespread muscle pain. This is evidenced by several attempts to create a unified theory of the origin of the FM and equally the development of reliable precise criteria for classification of FM, because of the existing classification based on the integration of different combinations of psycho-somatic disorders, based on a purely phenomenological approach, without taking into account the relationship and common pathogenic mechanisms of development and progression [8–10].

2. Aims of study

Given the extreme heterogeneity of clinical manifestations and the heterogeneity of quantitative measurements of different blood parameters, as well as a significant reduction in the quality of life in patients with FM, we set the main goal—the study of pathogenic features and diagnostic criteria as a basis for effective management of fibromyalgia. In accordance with the purpose, the following tasks were formulated:

—to examine the severity of the main clinical symptoms of FM, especially their relationships depending on the duration of the disease;

—to assess the level of physical and mental components of quality of life and the nature of their relationship with the symptoms of FM;

—to identify the role of pain, sleep disorders, duration of the disease as risk factors for developing depression in patients with FM.

3. Study design

The material of the study is based on 151 patients with verified diagnosis of FM; average age of the patients is 49.8 ± 13.3 years (M ± SD): among 129 women, average age is 49.7 ± 13.7 years, and 22 men, average age is 50.1 ± 5 years; the ratio of women to men is about 6:1. The average duration of the disease in patients with FM, regardless of age and sex, was 4.5 ± 2.4 years (M ± SD). FM patients with typical complains to persistent pain, poor sleep, chronic fatigue, general weakness, forgetfulness, and emotional instability were screened.

Inclusion criteria: The presence of pain at 11 tender points or more, negative rheumatology, age over 10 up to 79 years.

Exclusion criteria: Positive rheumatology, the presence of comorbidity with verified diagnosis of multiple sclerosis, diabetes, cancer, alcoholic neuropathy—diseases that are characterized by a poly-neuropathic pain; the age of patients—younger than 10 and older than 80 years due to allodynia, common in children and the elderly.

Type of study: From the perspective of evidence-based medicine, the study is observational, prospective, and noninvasive in nature. Due to study design no case-matching control group was selected and/or compared.

Research methods: The intensity of pain was assessed by visual analog scale (VAS) and the quality of sleep on a 10-point scale ("Questionnaire scoring subjective characteristics of sleep"). To identify the level of depressive symptoms all included in the study, patients with FM were evaluated by validated and standardized questionnaire Beck Depression Inventory (BDI) [11], which allows differentiating both the low level of depression and major depression. Total score in points is as follows: (0–9) the absence of depression, (10–25) low level of depression, and (26–39) major depression.

To examine the risk factors in patients with FM were used conventional relative risks: odds ratio (OR) and relative risk (RR)—the ratio of the probability (chance) events in the same group to the probability of an event in another group. OR and RR values between 0 and 1.0 correspond to the reduction in risk, >1.0 an increase in the relative risk [12–14].

The quality of life of patients was assessed by a questionnaire SF-36 HRQOL (v.2) [12, 15]. The latter consists of 11 questions, including 36 points, each of which has own set of positive symptoms and denies the allegations. The SF-36 application is mostly justified by the opportunity to assess the overall quality of life and its physical and mental components.

Ethic regulations: Inclusion of patients to the study was done with their informed consent. The ethical aspect of the study was reviewed by the Committee on Bioethics of Yerevan State Medical University; decision was made to comply with the requirements of relevant studies required for ethical standards.

The evaluation of the statistical significance of differences in the studied parameters was carried out by student's t-criterion. Statistical analysis was performed using software packages STATISTICA 6, GraphPad Prism 4, and GraphPad Prism 5. When carrying out the statistical analysis, follow the guidelines by Rosner [16] and De Muth [17].

4. Quantification of the major clinical symptoms of fibromyalgia and their relationship

4.1. Pain symptom evaluation

Test results on VAS show that in the total sample of patients with FM, pain intensity in the range of 1–5 points (4.9 ± 0.25, M ± SE) was detected in 37.1% of patients and 10.6 points (7.1 ± 1.25) in 62.9% of patients. These values were 59.0 and 41.0% for men and among women, 33.3 and 66.7% (**Figure 1**).

The study on the severity of pain in patients with FM, depending on the duration of the disease, revealed approximately the same the percentage of cases with the intensity of pain more or <5

points on the VAS scale, 51.9 and 48.1%, respectively. The group of patients with disease duration of FM for 3–5 years, especially more than 5 years, have seen a progressive increase in the percentage of patients with pain intensity >5 points, respectively, to 64.1 and 73.5% (**Figure 2**).

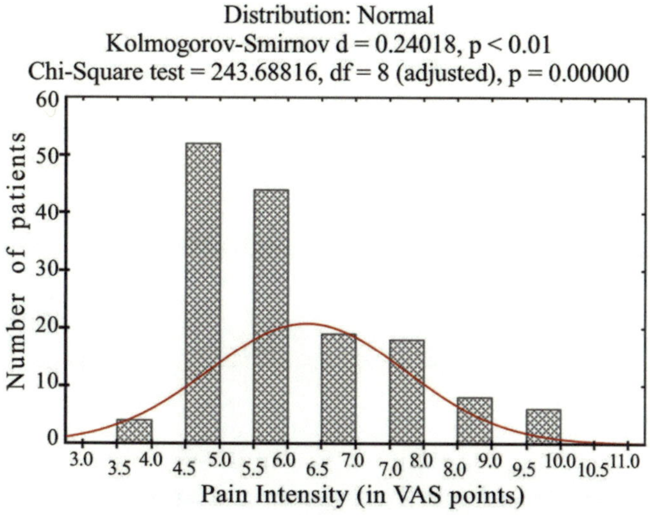

Figure 1. Results of the frequency distribution analysis indicator of the intensity of pain in the total sample of patients with FM.

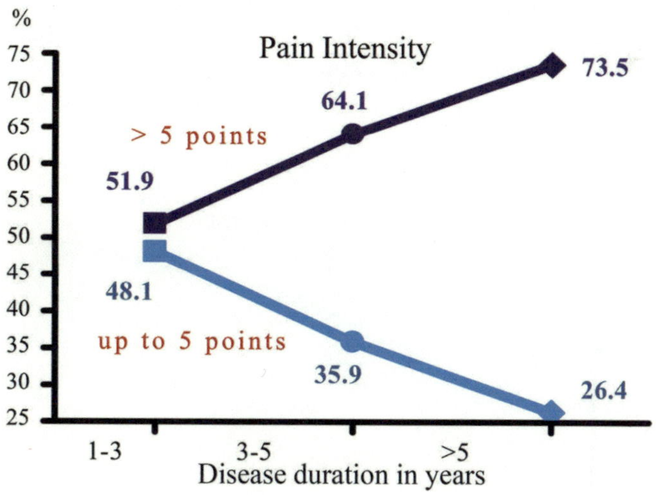

Figure 2. Intensity of pain in patients with FM, depending on the duration of the disease.

4.2. Sleep disorders

In the total sample of patients with FM, sleep disorders within 1–5 points (2.7 ± 0.13, M ± SE) were detected in 76.2% of patients and 6–10 points (6.5 ± 0.12) in 23.8% of patients, respectively, in men: 72.7 and 27.3% and in women: 33.3 and 66.7% (**Figure 3**).

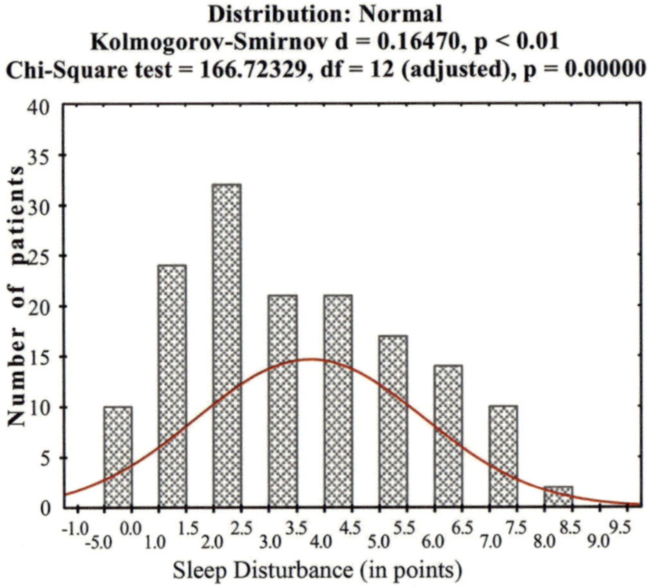

Figure 3. The results of frequency analysis of the distribution of index sleep disorders in the total sample of patients with FM.

It is well established that severity of sleep disorders is gradually reduced within the time-course of FM. For example, if a group of patients with disease duration of 1–3 years and the severity of sleep disorders <5 points found in 63.5% of cases, the duration of the disease for 3–5 years of the specified figure is 86.8% and more than 5 years is 97.8%. Against this background, notable decrease in the percentage of patients with severity of sleep disorders >5 points from 36.5 to 13.2% and 2.2% (**Figure 4**).

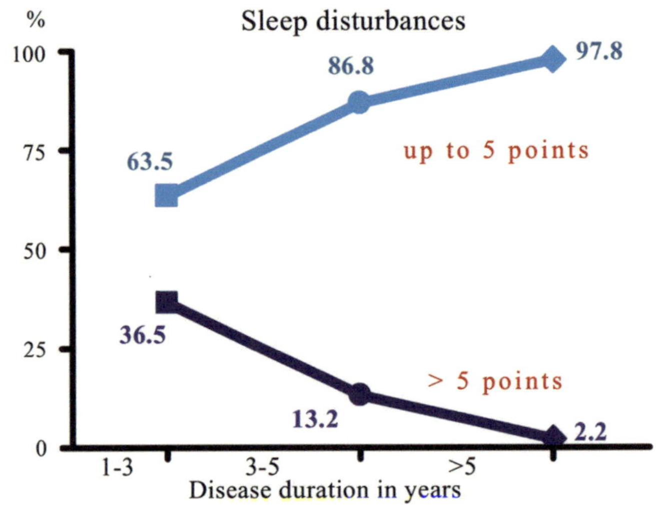

Figure 4. The severity of sleep disorders in patients with FM, depending on the duration of the disease.

http://dx.doi.org/10.5772/66671

These data coincidence with the recent results of Paul-Savoie [18] who believes that the role of deficiency of endogenous inhibitors of pain mechanisms and sleep disorder in the FM is quite polemical, and requires further analysis. Indeed, as evidenced by these data, indicators of the level of pain and sleep disorders in patients with common ferromagnetic sample are statistically significant negative correlation (**Figure 5**).

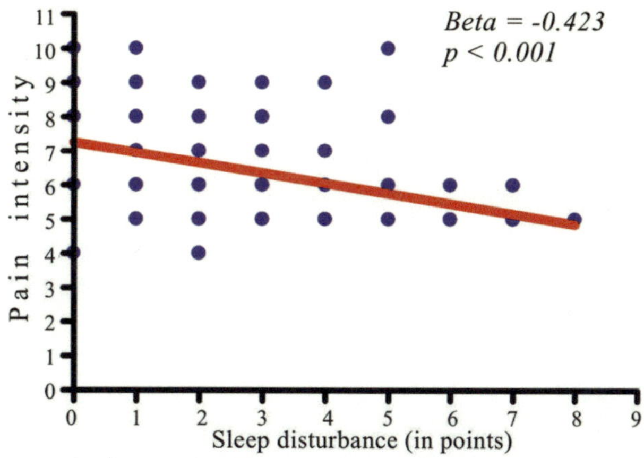

Figure 5. The relationship level of pain and sleep disorders in patients with FM.

4.3. Depressive symptoms

The Beck Depression Inventory questionnaire in patients, included in this study, found that the number of examinees with FM in 86.8% of cases has positive depressive symptoms and the absence of depression at 13.2% of patients. The severity of depressive symptoms in the group of positive patients was distributed as mild level of depression in 54.9% of detected cases and 45.1% of major depression (**Figures 6** and **7**).

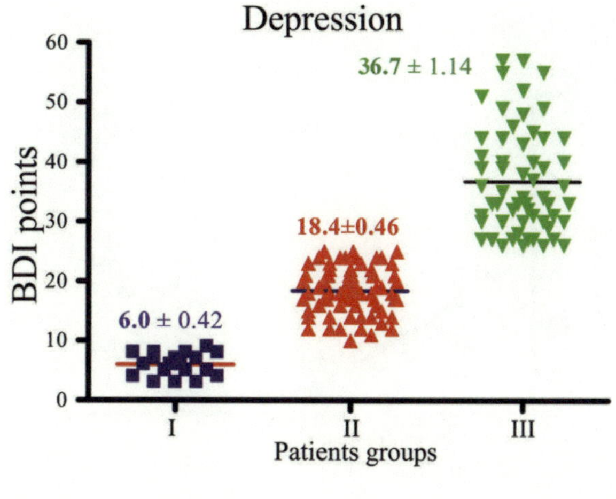

Figure 6. The test results of patients with FM on the depression scale BDI. Legend: *I*no signs of depression, *II*light level of depression, and *III*-major depression.

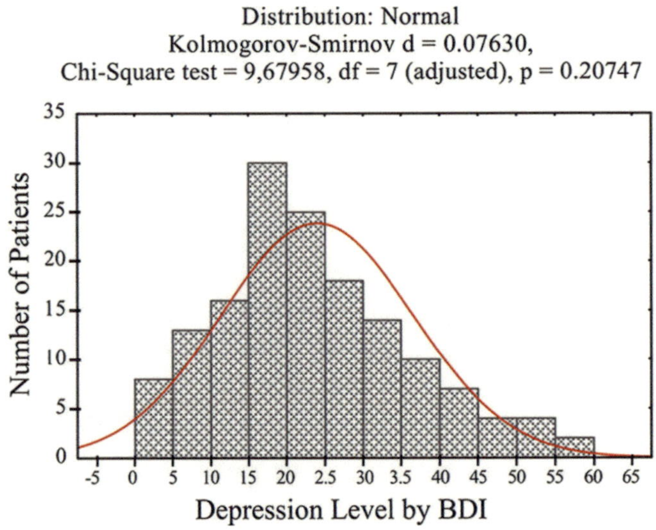

Figure 7. Frequency distribution of the index level of depression in the total sample of patients with FM.

These findings are consistent with the results of a number of authors, according to which the depressive disorders were observed in approximately 90% of patients with FM and major depression was established in 62–86% of cases [12, 19–22].

It is well established that increasing the FM duration develops a sharp decrease in the percentage of patients with no signs of depression, while drawn to that of patients with a disease duration of more than 5 years there has been a sharp increase in the percentage of patients with major depression symptoms that occur due to reduction in the specific proportion of patients with moderate depression (**Figure 8**).

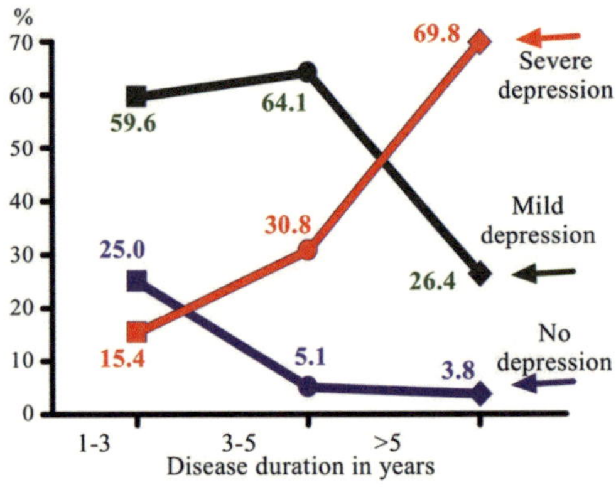

Figure 8. Dynamics of changes in the structure of depressive symptoms depending on the duration of the disease.

Thus, it should be regarded as established that increasing the duration of the disease in patients with FM observed parallelism in an escalation of depression and the severity of pain syndrome, which is accompanied by a reduction in the index of severity of sleep disorders.

At the same time, the data revealed that the rate of depressive mood in FM was significantly positively correlated with the indicator of the level of pain (r = 0.725, P < 0.0001) and negatively with the exponent of sleep disorders (r = -0.631, P < 0.001) (**Figure 9**).

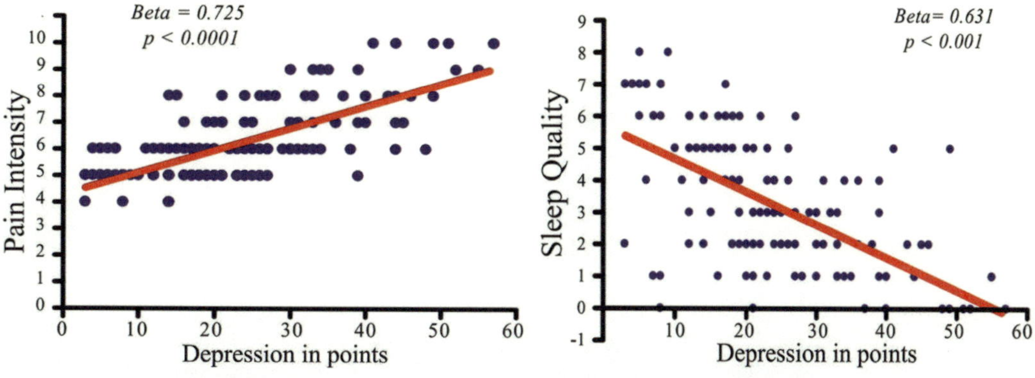

Figure 9. The relationship of depression with indicators of the level of pain and the degree of sleep disorders.

It should be emphasized that correlation between depression and pain in FM must be regarded as certain fact, while numerous data suggest that underlying pain symptoms and depression in FM share common pathogenic mechanisms [22–25]. Taking into account that according to the test results, using Beck Depression Inventory questionnaire in the studied sample of patients identified in 45.1% of major depression (according to DSM-IVTM ICD-9-CM Codes), with the aim of studying the role of pain symptoms, sleep disorders, and disease duration in the development of major depression in the FM calculated indicators such as the relative risk odds ratio (OR) and relative risk (RR). OR and RR values between 0 and 1.0 correspond to the reduction and >1.0 increase in the relative risk [13, 14].

The results of these studies suggest that the relative risk of major depression in patients with FM in the pain intensity in the range of 1–5 points is significantly lower (OR = 0.119, RR = 0.182) than at the level of pain >5 points (OR = 0.830, RR = 0.889), although in both cases they are lower than in the total sample. It is noteworthy that increasing the duration of the disease in patients with FM marked increase in the risk of developing major depression. So, if patients with a disease duration of FM for 1–3 years had OR = 0.283, RR = 0.393, and for 3–5 years had OR = 0.693, RR = 0.787, the relative risk of major depression in patients with "experience" of more than 5 years increases dramatically: OR = 3.577, RR = 1.782.

Enough interesting pattern is revealed in the study of the role of sleep disorders as a relative risk factor for major depression. As evidenced by the data presented, the relative risk of major depression revealed the severity of sleep disorders in the 1–3 score (OR = 1.871, RR = 1.396), whereas, in sleep disorders exceeding 3 points, relative risk is lower than for the total sample, accounting at 3–5 points: OR = 0.415, RR = 0.538 and >5 points: OR = 0.129, RR = 0.196 (**Table 1**).

Indicators	OR	RR	SS	SP
	Pain intensity			
1–5 points	0.119*** 0.041 ÷ 0.349	0.182*** 0.069 ÷ 0.480	0.063 0.017 ÷ 0.154	0.638 0.554 ÷ 0.717
>5 points	0.830* 0.486 ÷ 1.416	0.889* 0.632 ÷ 1.249	0.358 0.261 ÷ 0.465	0.597 0.515 ÷ 0.675
	Disease duration			
1–3 years	0.283** 0.124 ÷ 0.644	0.393** 0.201 ÷ 0.767	0.119 0.052 ÷ 0.221	0.676 0.591 ÷ 0.754
3–5 years	0.693* 0.325 ÷ 1.474	0.787* 0.472 ÷ 1.313	0.169 0.090 ÷ 0.276	0.773 0.687 ÷ 0.844
>5 years	3.577*** 1.855 ÷ 6.900	1.782*** 1.369 ÷ 2.320	0.398 0.300 ÷ 0.501	0.844 0.762 ÷ 0.906
	Sleep disturbances			
1–3 points	1.871* 1.074 ÷ 3.260	1.396* 1.050 ÷ 1.857	0.415 0.318 ÷ 0.518	0.724 0.638 ÷ 0.799
3–5 points	0.415* 0.178 ÷ 0.968	0.538* 0.282 ÷ 1.029	0.119 0.052 ÷ 0.228	0.754 0.667 ÷ 0.827
>5 points	0.129** 0.029–0.570	0.196** 0.051–0.756	0.032 0.051–0.756	0.793 0.708–0.862

*P < 0.05,
**P < 0.01,
***P < 0.001.

Table 1. Characteristics of relative risk factors in patients with major depression FM. Designations: OR, odds ratio; RR, relative risk; SS, sensitivity; SP, specificity.

Over the past decade has been widely used the term "quality of life" (QoL), which was acquired as interdisciplinary concept, an area of interest of researchers representing different industries and medical societies. It has turned scientific mind in the 1960s as a reaction to the dominance of objective indicators for assessing the usefulness of life factors such as income level, disease, and others. In contrast to objective criteria, the development and use of indicators of subjective well-being were needed. The term "quality of life," which, in the medical literature, is actually first used by Elkinton [26], is currently in the focus of researchers and is widely used in all the areas of clinical medicine.

Given that the polymorphism of the pathogenesis of FM, as well as an escalation in patients with signs of psycho-somatization, domestic and psychosocial maladjustment, induced spectrum of stressful factors, along with the monitoring of the main clinical symptoms of the disease and, especially, depression, assessment of physical and mental components of QoL plays an important role. The basis of modern trends of the development of psychometric research on the principle of multimodality, involving a transition from uni-variant representations to the multi-variant approach, provides a wide variation in various individual categories including data plane, data sources, methods of inspection, and other constructs.

The terms "multimodality" and "constructs" meant that rational choice construct is defined by the current level of research, with the distinction of traditional constructs integrated in global constructs and multidimensional constructs; for example, the test is to assess the level of quality of life—health-related quality of life (HRQOL the SF-36)—by which the quality of life of patients with FM was studied.

The test results of patients with FM, regardless of age, gender, and duration of illness, revealed a reduced level of quality of life, and the reduction in its total level is equal to the result of a reduced level of physical and mental component of quality of life that is inherent mainly in psychosomatic pathology. Below are data from a study of various indicators of the quality of life of patients with FM which show that the lowest levels are detected on the scale of physical activity, physical pain, emotional factor, and psychic health (**Figures 10** and **11**).

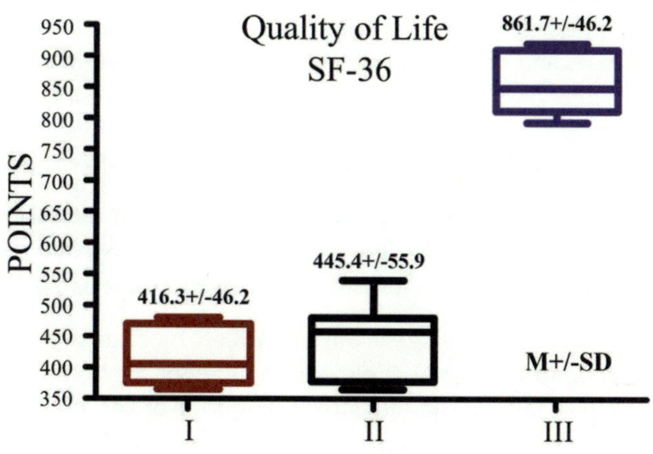

Figure 10. The physical (and) mental (II) components and total level (III) QoL FM (based on the SF-36).

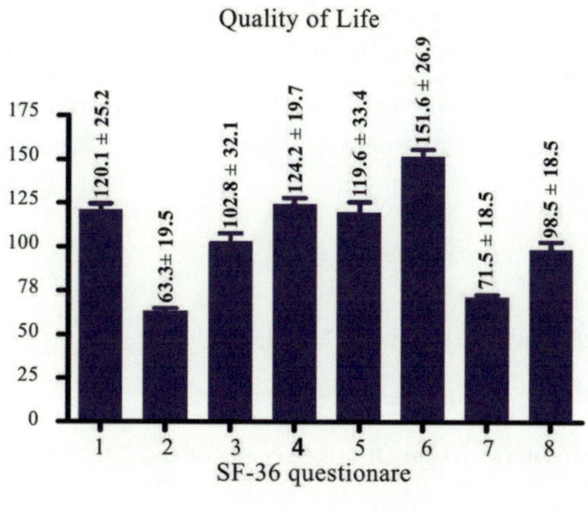

Figure 11. The level of various indicators of quality of life of patients with FM. Legend: *1* physical condition, physical activity *2*, *3*, physical pain, general health, *4*, *5*, vitality, social activity of *6* and *7* emotional factor, *8* mental health (by the SF-36).

Nonparametric correlation method was studied in patients with FM correlated with indicators of depression and quality of life scales. Studies conducted with the help of SF-36 indicate a negative, statistically significant correlation of depression not only with mental ($r = -0.663$, $P < 0.001$), but also with the physical component ($r = -0.447$) as well as with the total level of QOL ($r = -0.548$, $P < 0.001$). It is essential to identify the highest rates of negative correlation of depression with different indices of SF-36 scale with the "viability" ($r = -0.613$, $P < 0.001$).

5. Conclusion

As it is well known, the study of various aspects of FM, almost the same diagnostic criterion and the target of pharmacological intervention, is depression. Considering that depressive symptoms were detected in 86.8% of patients suffering from FM, special attention was paid to the study of major depression (according to DSM-IV "major depression"), which is found in patients in 45.1% of cases and occurs almost twice as likely to have women, which is comparable with those of a number of authors. Presented published data together with the results of this study convincingly show highly informative indicators of physical and mental components of quality of life, especially in the study of various aspects of FM and depression.

This approach was dictated by the fact that in many cases, major depressive signs, acting as dominant clinical manifestations of FM, are characterized by severe symptoms and high risk of suicides in this connection; the group of patients needs more specialized mental healthcare.

Similar humoral and neuronal pathogenically identified mechanisms trigger the development of both FM and depression, and clinical investigations pronounced the correlation of depression with pain, proving the fact that after a diagnosis of FM, quantitative indicators of depression and pain, along with an assessment of indicators of physical and mental components of QoL, become reliable criterion for efficacy of treatment and follow-up monitoring of the disease. It also must be considered that exacerbation of the chronic pain with depressive symptoms could lead to severe incapability and temporary disability, worsening the condition and chances to better outcomes. Those patients need more both medical and social attention, which finally increases the costs of treatment and burden to society.

Current effective treatment of chronic pain must refer to the presence and severity of depression, and depression effective management must include pain control therapies as well.

Author details

Aleksandra A. Karapetyan and Hovhannes M. Manvelyan*

*Address all correspondence to: manvelian@yahoo.com

Department of Family Medicine, Department of Neurology, Yerevan State Medical University, Yerevan, Armenia

http://dx.doi.org/10.5772/66671

References

[1] Baldry P.E. Myofascial Pain and Fibromyalgia Syndromes: A Clinical Guide to Diagnosis and Management. New York: Churchill-Livingstone. 2001.

[2] Wolfe F., Häuser W. Fibromyalgia diagnosis and diagnostic criteria. Ann Med. 2011; 43(7): 495–502.

[3] Kingsley J.D. Autonomic dysfunction in women with fibromyalgia. Arthritis Res Ther. 2012; 14(1): 103.

[4] Arnold L.M., Hudson J.I., Hess E.V., Ware A.E., Fritz D.A., et al. Family study of fibromyalgia. Arthritis Rheum. 2004; 50(3): 944–952.

[5] Blankfield A.A. Brief historic overview of clinical disorders associated with tryptophan: the relevance to chronic fatigue syndrome (CFS) and fibromyalgia (FM). Int J Tryptophan Res. 2012; 5: 27–32.

[6] Goldenberg D.L., Clauw D.J., Fitzcharles M.A. New concepts in pain research and pain management of the rheumatic diseases. Semin Arthritis Rheum. 2011; 41: 319–334.

[7] Joustra M.L., Janssens K.A., Bültmann U., Rosmalen J.G. Functional limitations in functional somatic syndromes and well-defined medical diseases. Results from the general population cohort Life Lines. J Psychosom Res. 2015; 79(2): 94–99.

[8] Giesecke T., Williams D.A., Harris R.E., Cupps T.R., Tian X., et al. Subgrouping of fibromyalgia patients on the basis of pressure-pain threshold and psychological factors. Arthritis Rheum. 2003; 48(10): 2916–2922.

[9] Thieme K., Turk D.C., Flor H. Comorbid depression and anxiety in fibromyalgia syndrome: relationship to somatic and psychosocial variables. Psychosom Med. 2004; 66: 837–844.

[10] Müller W., Schneider E.M., Stratz T. The classification of fibromyalgia syndrome. Rheumatol Int. 2007; 27(11): 1005–1010.

[11] Beck A.T., Steer R.A., Brown G.K. Beck Depression Inventory. 2nd ed. San Antonio: The Psychological Corporation. 1996.

[12] Aguglia A., Salvi V., Maina G., Rossetto I., Aguglia E. Fibromyalgia syndrome and depressive symptoms: comorbidity and clinical correlates. J Affect Disord. 2011; 128(3): 262–266.

[13] Robbins A.S., Chao S.Y., Fonseca V.P. What's the relative risk? A method to directly estimate risk ratios in cohort studies of common outcomes. Ann Epidemiol. 2002; 12: 452–454.

[14] Viera A.J. Odds ratios and risk ratios: what's the difference and why does it matter? South Med J. 2008; 101(7): 730–734.

[15] Ware J.E., Kosinski M., Keller S.K. SF-36® Physical and Mental Health Summary Scales: A User's Manual. Boston, MA: The Health Institute. 1994.

[16] http://www.worldcat.org/title/fundamentals-of-biostatistics/oclc/32679234/editions?start_edition=21&sd=desc&referer=di&se=yr&editionsView=true&fq=ln%3Aeng.

[17] De Muth J.E. Overview of biostatistics used in clinical research. Am J Health-Syst Pharm. 2009; 66: 70–81.

[18] Paul-Savoie E., Marchand S., Morin M., Bourgault P., Brissette N., et al. Is the deficit in pain inhibition in fibromyalgia influenced by sleep impairments? Open Rheumatol J. 2012; 6: 296–302.

[19] Arnold L.M., Hudson J.I., Hess E.V. Family study of fibromyalgia. J Arthritis Rheum. 2004; 50: 944–952.

[20] Arnold L.M., Clauw D.J., Dunegan L.J., Turk D.C. FibroCollaborative. A framework for fibromyalgia management for primary care providers. Mayo Clin Proc. 2012; 87: 488–496.

[21] Maletic V., Raison C.L. Neurobiology of depression, fibromyalgia and neuropathic pain. Front Biosci. 2009; 14: 5291–5338.

[22] Marangell L.B., Clauw D.J., Choy E., Wang F., Shoemaker S., et al. Comparative pain and mood effects in patients with comorbid fibromyalgia and major depressive disorder: secondary analyses of four pooled randomized controlled trials of duloxetine. Pain. 2011; 152: 31–37.

[23] Williams L.J., Jacka F.N., Pasco J.A., Dodd S., Berk M. Depression and pain: an overview. Acta Neuropsychiatr. 2006; 18(2): 79–87.

[24] Bigatti S.M., Hernandez A.M., Cronan T.A., Rand K.L. Sleep disturbance in fibromyalgia syndrome: relationship to pain and depression. Arthritis Rheum. 2008; 59: 961–967.

[25] Ang D.C., Chakr R., France C.R., Mazzuca S.A., Stump T.E., et al. Association of nociceptive responsivity with clinical pain and the moderating effect of depression. J Pain. 2011; 12(3): 384–389.

[26] Elkinton J.R. Medicine and the quality of life. Ann Intern Med. 1966; 64(3): 711–714.

Section 3

The Proportion of Automatic Negative Thoughts and Selected Psychological Aspects Affecting the Development of Depression

Chapter 5

Investigating the Relationship between Depression, Negative Automatic Thoughts, Life Satisfaction and Symptom Interpretation in Turkish Young Adults

Yasemin Yavuzer and Zeynep Karataş

Additional information is available at the end of the chapter

http://dx.doi.org/10.5772/66622

Abstract

The purpose of this study is to examine the relationship between depression, negative automatic thoughts, life satisfaction, number of symptoms, psychologizing, somatizing and normalizing in young adults. The mediator role of life satisfaction in the relationship between negative automatic thoughts and depression especially is the major question of this study. Participants are composed of 115 volunteer teacher candidates from an urban Turkish university. Their ages vary between 21 and 29. The data are collected through Beck Depression Inventory, Life Satisfaction Scale, Automatic Thoughts Scale, Symptom Interpretation Questionnaire and Personal Information Form. As a result, it is seen that the depression scores of young adults do not differ according to gender and according to whether they encountered an event causing stress in the past 3 months or not. Another finding is that five variables (negative automatic thoughts, life satisfaction, number of symptoms, psychologizing and normalizing) are significant predictors in explaining the depression level of young adults. Together, these five variables explain 52% of the young adults' depression. Another finding of the study is that negative automatic thoughts of young adults make them negatively assess quality of life and this causes the depression levels to increase.

Keywords: automatic thoughts, life satisfaction, life events, symptom attribution type, depression, young adults

1. Introduction

Quality of life is a concept shaped by how an individual perceives his own life according to the society and culture he lives in. World Health Organization defines quality of life as the individual assessment of one's life positions in the context of their cultural and value systems in relation to their own personal goals, standards and concerns. This concept has a complex structure encompassing individual's physical health, psychological state, independence level, social relationships, personal beliefs, distinct characteristics and her relationship with the environment [1]. Quality of life is also defined as a concept affecting the level of personal satisfaction that can be achieved under living conditions and showing personal responses to sicknesses and physical, mental and social effects of daily life [2]. As is seen, however we define quality of life, it has a complex structure and mental state has an important part in this structure. In this study, variables like depression, negative automatic thoughts, life satisfaction that is a dimension of subjective well-being, attribution used by people to interpret physical symptoms and life events among the variables related to one's psychological state determining their quality of life and causing them to perceive their life as high-quality or poor-quality are examined.

1.1. Depression

Depression is common mental disorder among individuals that manifests itself as negative thoughts and frustration, despair and reluctance [3]. Although generally associated with feelings of sadness, being solely having feeling of sadness does not require clinical treatment of depression. Depression has a set of significant symptoms other than having feeling of sadness. These symptoms are emotional, cognitive, motivational and physical symptoms. While emotional symptoms manifest themselves as joylessness, loss of interest in normally enjoyable activities and low-self-esteem, cognitive symptoms manifest themselves as pessimism and despair. While motivational symptoms observed in depression can be explained by symptoms like indifference and weariness, physical symptoms presents themselves as difficulty in sleeping, loss of energy and appetite [4]. When theoretical structure related to depression is examined, according to Beck who states cognitive levels and thought processes as causal factors in depression, people with depression develop negative schemata as a result of parental loss, several consecutive tragedies, peer rejection and teacher criticism. Negative schemata or beliefs developed by people with depression activate when they encounter new events closely or remotely resembling the situations where they learned these schemata. Furthermore, negative schemata of depressed people awaken people's biases causing them to distort reality and these schemata are fueled by the aforementioned biases [5]. Beck's cognitive model asserts that depression arises from misinterpretation of one's experiences in a stubborn and negative way. These misinterpretations bring out a negative cognitive triad. This triad includes negative opinions of a person about himself, his world and his future. They see themselves as losers; they see the world as an environment including obstacles that prevents their satisfaction; and they believe that their future does not have any hope for their development [6]. Looking at the world with a negative perspective during the early childhood years teaches individuals to be disappointed. Focusing more on negative sides of the experienced events and life situations that are great sources of stress increase the risk of depression [7]. Depression can also be interpreted as learned helplessness where a person believes that the results of events cannot be controlled [7]. According to Seligman, the reason for depression is the belief that one cannot affect the events in his own life. By learning helplessness, the person believes that events are out of his control. According to behavior scientists, depression symptoms arise

http://dx.doi.org/10.5772/66622

from relationship problems with other people. The decrease in or loss of positive feedback from other people causes depression. If a person's behavior does not receive positive feedback from the others, this person becomes passive and introvert and shows cognitive symptoms of depression [8].

When studies related to depression are examined in the literature, it is seen that the rate of depression among women in developed countries is twice that of men [9]. The studies examining depression in terms of socioeconomic level and culture [10, 11] put forward that the rate of depression is higher at low socioeconomic level and there is a relation between depression and low socioeconomic level [9]. Also, in literature, there are studies examining cultural differences in depression in adults. While the studies showing there is no cultural difference in depression stand out among the studies in literature [12–14], the studies showing there is cultural difference in depression also stand out [15–24]. It was found in one of these studies examining depressive symptoms in Turkey and Canada that the level of depressive symptoms of the Turkish sample was higher than the Canadian sample [24]. In a study on depression using 967 university students from Australia, Iran and Portugal concluded that Australian students were more depressive compared to Iranian and Portuguese students and Iranian students were more depressive compared to Portuguese students [23]. A group of researchers studied depression among the Yoruba people, who are the largest of the three tribes in Nigeria, living in Nigerian countryside, Nigerian cities, Canadian countryside and American cities [22]. They concluded that depression was seen the lowest among the Yoruba living in the Nigerian countryside and the highest living in American cities. In another study, it was asked how they defined depression to the 110 English, South Asian and Caribbean participants in their study group and had found cultural differences [21]. In another research, the depression levels of Koreans, Korean Americans and Caucasian Americans were compared [20]. It was concluded that the depression levels of Koreans were higher compared to the other two groups. A group of researchers in Turkey compared Turkish patients diagnosed with depression living in Germany as migrants and Turkish patients diagnosed with depression living in Turkey [17]. They found that the migrant group's depression symptoms were higher. In another study it compared Turkish and German patients living in Germany and concluded that somatization was higher in Turks [15]. Chinese and American students' depression levels were examined and found that Chinese students' depression levels were significantly higher than American students' depression levels [18]. In a study [22] was compared depression levels in Turkish and English patients diagnosed with major depression and stated that while depressive mood, pessimism and loss of interest and enjoyment was prevalent in English patients, somatic anxiety was prevalent in Turkish patients [16].

1.2. Depression and negative automatic thoughts

Negative automatic thoughts are another important variable of depression. Negative automatic thoughts can be defined as an individual's statements about himself and inner talks with himself. These thoughts most often rise to the surface in certain affective disorders during the perceptions of the situations as a result of various cognitive distortions. The reason why these thoughts are identified as negative is because they cause besetting unpleasant emotions like sadness, guilt and anxiety [25]. Automatic thoughts form through schemas. Part of Beck's cognitive theory, schemas include the structural organization of thought or certain organized patterns. Schemas provide a basis for shaping cognition. The person evaluates the events, rules, or situations he faces through schemas or gives reactions appropriate to the schemas by reorganizing them. Even though past experiences are important in schemas, consistency in coding that schema is important. Schemas were used by Beck to explain why people with depression insist on hurtful behaviors while they defend themselves. Schemas, also, explain why depressive people generalize negative experiences, remember negative experiences, ignore positive experiences and see the negative experiences [26]. According to Beck, having a depressive schema makes people weak and vulnerable against depression. When depressive schema is active, automatic thoughts are produced in many ways and cognitive distortions are created. According to Beck, negative automatic thoughts are only characteristics of depressive situations. Depression is expressed as a more fundamental and more consistent cognitive weakness factor according to a depressive schema. Based on this model, it is more active in people who have more negative thoughts. This situation can disappear when the created schema becomes ineffective. A person's negative thoughts about himself and his future make them vulnerable against depression cognitively. The worse the depression is the higher the intensity of automatic thoughts. An increase in this kind of intensity in thoughts and a decrease in purposeful and logical thoughts causes depressive situation to increase [27].

1.3. Depression and life satisfaction

Life satisfaction is considered another variable that can be associated with depression. The greater the satisfaction the person gets from life, the stronger his hold on life and his enjoyment from life. When his life satisfaction is low, he will not enjoy life and he can show depressive symptoms. Life satisfaction is a cognitive part of subjective well-being. Thus, first there is need to understand the definition of subjective well-being.

Subjective well-being is a concept concerning with how people experience their lives affectively and cognitively [28] in a state where negative factors do not exist and positive cognitive and mental elements exist [29]. Individual's assessments include his emotional state, affective reactions toward events and judgments regarding life satisfaction. Subjective well-being is composed of three primary components. These components are: (1) cognitively assessing one's satisfaction he gets from life's private and general aspects (2) existence of positive affectivity and (3) lack of negative affectivity [30]. With the components of pleasant emotions, unpleasant emotions and life satisfaction, subjective well-being of people rises depending on the feeling of more pleasant emotions than unpleasant emotions and having positive cognitive judgment regarding their lives [31]. When life satisfaction and affectivity, components of subjective well-being, are examined, it can be said that life satisfaction is a person's subjective assessment of his quality of life and includes cognitive judgments about his own life. It is also a primary component of a person's subjective well-being [32]. In addition, it is stated that life satisfaction is closely related to morale, adjustment and psychological well-being [33]. Affectivity is associated with subjective well-being's affective aspect that includes mental state and emotions related to instantaneous events. While positive reaction to others and activities generally present pleasant affectivity, unpleasant affectivity includes negative reactions toward others in personal experiences. Emotions like anger, sadness, anxiety, worry, stress, disappointment, guilt, embarrassment, shame and envy underlie negative or unpleasant affectivity. Among the other negative affectivities [23], states like loneliness and helplessness are important symptoms of sickness. Some negative emotions are part of life and are effective in mobilizing individuals. However, observable and continuous negative affectivity can be symptoms of worsening in a person's life [34]. When primary components of subjective well-being explained by Diener et al. [35] are examined, it is seen that while emotions like joy, elation, contentment, pride, affection, happiness and ecstasy are discussed under the positive affect, emotions like guilt and shame, sadness, anxiety and worry, anger, stress, depression and envy are discussed under the negative affect. A person's life satisfaction includes desire to change life, satisfaction with current life, satisfaction with past, satisfaction with future and significant others' views of one's life. Satisfaction domains were grouped under work, family, leisure and health, finances, self and one's group. High subjective well-being of a person depends on that person increasing his satisfaction from life by using satisfaction domains in a healthy way, having more pleasant affects and reactions and less unpleasant affects and reactions.

Life satisfaction is a cognitive component of subjective well-being and is defined as assessment about one's own life [36, 37] and as positive assessment of one's whole life based on criteria determined by oneself [38]. Life satisfaction includes satisfaction from current life, desire to change life, satisfaction from past, satisfaction from future and significant others' views of one's life. Satisfaction domains are work, family, leisure, health, finances, self and one's close surroundings [39]. Life satisfaction is closely linked with psychological health. It is known that life satisfaction of people with good health is higher compared to people with bad health [40]. In the studies conducted, it is seen that people with high life satisfaction have more responsibility in their own different roles, have more satisfaction in romantic relations, school and family domains, have less stress [41] and less emotional loneliness [42], have higher self-esteem [43] and have lower depression, despair and anxiety levels [44]. Furthermore, it was determined that well-being of university students who receive adequate support from their parents and friends and who have positive thoughts about their own futures were higher [45].

1.4. Other variables related to depression

1.4.1. Stressful life events

Another variable related to depression is stressful life events. Traumatic life events, loops, losses, firsts and mosts generally have important place in a person's life. Traumatic life events are the most apparent important cause of psychological disorders. Traumatic life events include separation from parents, lover, spouse or friend, leaving the place he was born and raised or being taken away from that place, loosing loved ones, catching a mental or physical disease, experiencing violent events like war, torture, sexual harassment or rape, experiencing natural disasters like earthquake, flood, erosion and fire and professional, academic and business failures. These kinds of events are more likely to happen to psychiatric patients compared to people who are not sick [46]. Traumatic life events decrease a person's resistance by disturbing the mental balance of that person and make him prone to psychological disorders [46]. However, just like not everybody experiencing bad events do not develop psychiatric disorders, it is known that many people experiencing bad events do not kill themselves. Therefore, it is stressed that what leads people to kill themselves or to think about killing themselves is not the traumatic events but their strength and skills to cope with these events [47].

1.4.2. Somatic symptoms

Accepted as a factor that makes recognition of depression difficult, somatization is closely related to how a person interprets the physical symptoms he is experiencing and to what he connects them to [48]. According to Robbins and Kirmayer [49], when a person experiences minor physical symptoms, he normalizes them by attributing them to situational conditions like insomnia, eating irregularities, fatigue and environmental stimuli or he perceives them as pathological by attributing them to abnormal mental and physical conditions. Although somatization is associated with various psychiatric disorders, it is mostly known to accompany depression and anxiety disorders. Physical complaints may be the foremost signs of depression. Body aches and pains, intestinal disorders and digestive problems are common [50]. It is argued that 10–30% of psychiatric inpatients and outpatients diagnosed with depression complained about physical symptoms [51]. Since young adulthood represents entrance to adulthood, it is one of the most important turning points in a person's life. During young adulthood, individuals have developmental tasks like spouse selection, learning to live with the spouse, having a family, raising a child, developing career by entering a job, assuming citizenship responsibilities and joining an appropriate social group. It is stated that the most important threat during the first years of adulthood is not to be able to build close and deep relationships and become isolated [52]. Thus, this period is a period when young adults encounter social and physical changes, face many emotional, behavioral, sexual, economic, academic and social conflicts and increase their effort to find their identity with psychosocial and sexual maturity. It is reported that 62% of the university students consult psychological counseling services about depressive symptoms [53]. Depression in adolescents is one of the most common mental disorders that cause serious disruptions in psychosocial and academic functions and to prevent overcoming developmental problems [54]. Therefore, the purpose of this study is to examine the relationship between depression, negative automatic thoughts, life satisfaction, number of symptoms, psychologizing, somatizing and normalizing in young adults. The mediator role of life satisfaction in the relationship between negative automatic thoughts and depression especially is the major question of this study.

2. Method

2.1. Research design and participants

This is a correlational and quantitative research aiming to examine the relations of depression with automatic thoughts, life satisfaction, number of symptoms, psychologizing, somatizing and normalizing in young adults. Participants are composed of 115 volunteer teacher candidates from an urban Turkish university. Whereas 100 of the participants (46.5%) are female, the remaining 115 (53.5%) are male. Their ages vary between 21 and 29 (Mean ± SD = 24.41 ± 3.04). While 164 (76.3%) of the participants stated that they encountered an event causing stress during the past 3 months, 51 (23.7%) of them stated that they did not encounter an event causing stress during the past 3 months. Thirty four (15.8%) of the 164 participants who stated that they encountered an event causing stress during the past 3 months had health-related problems. Twenty four (11.2%) of them had family-related problems; 25 (11.6%) had problems related to romantic relationships; 13 (6%) had problems with their friends; 11 (5.1%) had school-related problems; and 22 (10.2%) had financial problems. Nineteen (8.8%) of them lost someone close and 16 (7.4%) of them stated that they experienced events like custody or arrest.

2.2. Data collection instruments

Personal Information Form: In the Personal Information Form, the participants were asked about their gender, age and whether they encountered an event causing stress during the past 3 months or not and what kind of event it was.

Beck Depression Inventory (BDI): The inventory, developed by Beck et al. and adapted to Turkish by Hisli [55] has 21 items. There are four subscales (impairment in performance, negative feelings toward one's self, somatic disorders and feeling guilty). Total scores were used in the present study. It was reported that split-half reliability of the scale was 0.74 and criterion-dependent validity was 0.63. Internal consistency coefficient of the scale was 0.80 for this study [55].

Life Satisfaction Scale (LSS): Diener et al. [38] developed the scale and it was adapted to Turkish by Köker [56] and Yetim [57]. The scale is a 7-point Likert-type self-report scale ranging from "Does not apply at all (1)" to "completely applies (7)." It was found that test retest reliability of the scale, which was carried out with 3-week interval, was 0.85. In the present study, internal consistency coefficient of LSS was 0.82 [56].

Automatic Thoughts Scale (ATS): The 30-item 5-point Likert-type ATS was scale developed by Hollan and Kendall [58] and adapted for use in Turkey by Şahin and Şahin [59]. The minimum score is 30 and the maximum score is 150. Higher scores indicate a higher frequency of automatic thoughts. Research on the reliability of the Turkish version calculated its Cronbach's alpha internal consistency coefficient as 0.93. The item total correlations between item scores and total score were calculated as 0.30–0.69 [60]. In the present study the internal reliability was calculated as 0.87. The ATS was developed to identify automatic thoughts associated with depression.

Symptom Interpretation Questionnaire (SIQ): It is a self-report measure that assesses how people interpret common physical symptoms. Respondents are asked to interpret 13 common physical symptoms as either somatizing (physical disorder), psychologizing (emotional distress), or normalizing (normal environmental event) by grading. It was developed by Robbins and Kirmayer [49] and its validity and reliability study was conducted by Duman et al. [48]. The scale was turned into a 5-point Likert-type scale in its Turkish version. Addition of the 14 question to the scale is the second change made to the scale. According to the scale's subscales, internal consistency coefficient was calculated as 0.87 for somatizing, 0.87 for psychologizing and 0.86 for normalizing.

2.3. Data analysis

Data was analyzed using SPSS v.22.0 for Windows. T-test was used for the examination of the effect of gender and the life events on DS, ATS, SIQ subscales scores and LSS scores. Simple and hierarchical multiple linear regression analyses were used to analyze the data. Before conducting the analyses, assumptions of the multiple linear regressions were tested. It was determined that normality and linearity assumptions of the multiple linear regressions were satisfied. Before analyses, conformity of the data to normal distribution was tested by looking at its skewness and kurtosis values. Skewness values were between 1.06 and −0.45 and kurtosis values were between −0.72 and 1.18. Skewness and kurtosis values should ideally be between +1 and −1 but values between +2 and −2 are considered as acceptable [61]. When testing autocorrelation, the Durbin-Watson coefficient was used. Durbin-Watson values varied between 1.78 and 1.97. Tolerance and VIF values were also within acceptable limits. In addition, as reported in the methodological literature, correlation coefficients between predictor variables that are 0.90 or above [62] or 0.80 or above [63] indicate a multicollinearity problem. In this study, correlation coefficients between predictor variables varied between −0.02 and 0.72. In the present study, mediator role of life satisfaction in the relationship between automatic thoughts and depression was investigated by using Pearson correlation coefficient, simple and multiple linear regression based on Baron and Kenny's [64] proposed conditions. Conditions are as follows: (1) two variables – depression and automatic thoughts should be significantly correlated. (2) suggested mediator variable–life satisfaction–should be correlated with these two variables and (3) when mediator variable had controlled the correlation between the two variables should diminish. The significance of the decay between Beta (β) values were analyzed by using the Sobel test.

3. Results

3.1. Examination of the difference of gender and the stressful life events on DS, ATS, SIQ subscales scores and LSS scores

The findings showed that there were significant gender-based differences in SIQ NS ($t = 2.64$, $p < 0.001$) P ($t = 3.05$, $p < 0.001$) subscale scores and LSS ($t = 2.50$, $p < 0.01$) scores, but not in the DS ($t = 1.39$, $p > 0.05$), ATS ($t = -0.03$, $p > 0.05$) scores and SIQ S ($t = 1.67$, $p > 0.05$), N ($t = 0.57$, $p > 0.05$) subscales scores. These findings indicate that the females had higher SIQ NS and *P* subscale scores and LSS scores than did the males (**Table 1**). Another finding is that there were significant differences in SIQ NS ($t = 2.29$, $p < 0.01$) subscale scores based on whether the student encountered an event causing stress during the past 3 months. This result shows that the students who encountered an event causing stress during the past 3 months had higher SIQ NS subscale scores than did the students who did not encountered an event causing stress during the past 3 months (**Table 1**).

3.2. The relationships between the study variables

The Pearson product-moment correlation technique was used to explain the relationships between the study variables. The relationships between the study variables, mean values and SDs of the variables are shown in **Table 2**. The findings showed that there were positive correlations between the students' DS and ATS scores ($r = 0.65$, $p < 0.01$), between DS and SIQ NS subscale scores ($r = 0.24$, $p < 0.01$), between DS and SIQ P subscale scores ($r = 0.47$, $p < 0.01$), between DS and SIQ S subscale scores ($r = 0.32$, $p < 0.01$), between DS and SIQ N subscale scores ($r = 0.17$, $p < 0.05$). There was also a negative correlation between the students' DS and LSS scores ($r = 0.50$, $p < 0.01$). Furthermore, it was found that there was no significant relationship between DS scores and age and stressful life event.

	Gender				
	Male ($n = 115$)		Female ($n = 100$)		
	M	*SD*	*M*	*SD*	*t*
Depression Scale	14.62	8.44	16.31	9.23	1.39
Automatic Thoughts Scale	64.60	21.31	65.52	20.22	-0.03
SIQ subscales					
Number of symptoms	7.67	4.05	9.02	3.27	2.64*
Psychologizing	32.16	10.24	36.91	12.52	3.05*
Somatizing	29.61	9.38	31.92	10.79	1.67
Normalizing	34.95	10.21	35.79	11.18	0.57
Life Satisfaction Scale	21.20	6.84	23.39	5.75	2.50*
Did you encounter an event causing stress during the past 3 months?					
	Yes ($n = 164$)		**No ($n = 51$)**		
	M	**SD**	**M**	**SD**	**t**
Depression Scale	15.98	8.86	13.58	8.62	1.69
Automatic Thoughts Scale	64.63	19.86	64.35	23.66	0.08
SIQ subscales					
Number of symptoms	8.62	3.67	7.25	3.90	2.29*
Psychologizing	35.12	11.99	31.94	9.85	1.72
Somatizing	31.20	10.33	29.01	9.21	1.35
Normalizing	35.97	10.71	33.31	10.31	1.56
Life Satisfaction Scale	21.87	6.63	23.33	5.69	1.41

SIQ, Symptom Interpretation Questionnaire, *p < 0.01.

Table 1. The effect of gender and the life events on DS, ATS, SIQ sub scales scores and LSS scores.

			SIQ sub scales									
	M	SD	DS	ATS	NS	P	S	N	LSS	AGE	LE
DS	15.41	8.84	1.00								
ATS	64.56	20.79	0.65**	1.00							
SIQ subscales											
NS	8.30	3.76	0.24**	0.11	1.00						
P	34.37	11.58	0.47**	0.47**	0.48**	1.00					
S	30.68	10.10	0.32**	0.34**	0.39**	0.70**	1.00				
N	35.34	10.66	0.17*	0.23**	0.28**	0.65**	0.72**	1.00			
LSS	22.22	6.43	−0.50**	−0.48**	−0.13	−0.33**	−0.23**	−0.18**	1.00		
AGE	24.41	3.84	−0.08	−0.10	−0.16*	−0.19**	−0.20**	−0.22**	−0.02	1.00	
LE	0.79	0.42	0.12	0.00	0.16*	0.12	0.09	0.11	−0.09	0.00	1.00

DS, Depression Scale; ATS, Automatic Thoughts Scale; SIQ, Symptom Interpretation Questionnaire; NS, number of symptoms; P, psychologizing; S =somatizing; N, normalizing; LSS, Life Satisfaction Scale; LE, stressful life event, *p < 0.05, **p < 0.01.

Table 2. The relationships between the study variables and their mean ± SDs.

3.3. Predictors of depression

Predictors of depression were examined in six steps using hierarchical multiple regression analysis to consider the correlation coefficients between variables. Gender, age and stressful life event were not included in the regression analysis since they did not create a difference in DS scores and since they were not related to DS scores. The first step evaluated automatic thoughts; the second step life satisfaction; the third step number of symptoms; the fourth step psychologizing; the fifth step somatizing; and the last step normalizing. The analysis results are shown in **Table 3**.

Table 3 shows that five variables (ATS, LSS, SIQ NS, P and N subscales) are significant predictors in explaining the depression level of young adults. The results of the first step of analysis indicate that automatic thoughts had a significant effect ($\beta = 0.65$, $p < 0.01$). The findings also show that automatic thoughts scores account for 42% of the total variance in young adults' depression levels. Furthermore, it appears that the contribution of the life satisfaction entered in the second step of the model was significant ($\beta = -0.24$, $p < 0.01$), accounting for 5% of variance related to depression. Together, these two variables explain 47% of the young adults' depression. The results of the third step of analysis indicate that number of symptoms had a significant effect ($\beta = 0.15$, $p < 0.01$) and explained 2% of the variance. Together, these three variables explain 49% of the young adults' depression. The contribution of the psychologizing entered in the fourth step of the model was significant ($\beta = 0.13$, $p < 0.05$) and explained 1% of the variance. Together, these four variables explain 50% of the young adults' depression. On the other hand, it appears that somatizing, entered in the fifth step, was not a significant predictor ($\beta = -0.05$, $p > 0.05$). It is found that normalizing, which was entered in the last step, was a significant predictor ($\beta = -0.19$, $p < 0.05$) and explained 2% of the variance. Together, these five variables explain 52% of the young adults' depression.

Model	Independent variables	β	t	R^2	R^2_{ch}	F_{ch}
1	ATS	0.65	12.49**	0.42	0.42	156.20**
2	LSS	−0.24	−4.22**	0.47	0.05	17.83**
3	NS	0.15	3.06**	0.49	0.02	9.40**
4	P	0.13	2.08*	0.50	0.01	4.34*
5	S	−0.05	−0.79	0.50	0.00	0.62
6	N	−0.19	−2.53*	0.52	0.02	6.42*

ATS, Automatic Thoughts Scale; LSS , Life Satisfaction Scale; NS, number of symptoms; P, psychologizing; S, somatizing; N, normalizing, *p < 0.05, **p < 0.01.

Table 3. Hierarchical multiple regression analysis results related to predicting young adults' depression scale scores.

3.4. Mediating test results

Regression analysis of the mediating role of life satisfaction in the relationship between automatic thoughts and depression was conducted in three steps [64]. The findings are shown in **Table 4**.

In the first step, automatic thoughts positively and significantly predicted depression ($\beta = 0.65$, $p < 0.001$) and explained 42% of the variation. In the second step automatic thoughts negatively and significantly predicted life satisfaction ($\beta = -0.48$, $p < 0.001$) and explained 23% of the variance. In the third step, life satisfaction was identified as a mediating variable that negatively and significantly predicted depression ($\beta = -0.24$, $p < 0.001$). Life satisfaction and automatic thoughts together explained 47% of the variance. In the third step, it was observed that taken together with the mediator variable (LSS), there was a reduction in the strength of the correlation between the ATS and the DS (see **Table 4**). These findings indicate that LSS partially mediated the relationship between ATS and DS for the young adults (Sobel $z = 3.99$, $p < 0.001$).

	Variables	β	t
Step 1	ATS	0.65**	12.49**
(DS/dependent variable)	$R = 0.65$, $R^2 = 0.42$, $F = 156.20$**		
Step 2	ATS	−0.48	−7.87**
(LSS/Dependent variable)	$R = 0.48$, $R^2 = 0.23$, $F = 61.99$**		
Step 3	ATS	0.53**	9.42**
(DS/Dependent variable)	LSS	−0.24	−4.22**
	$R = 0.69$, $R^2 = 0.47$, $F = 93.21$**		

DS, Depression Scale; ATS, Automatic Thoughts Scale; LSS, Life Satisfaction Scale, **p < 0.001.

Table 4. Regression analysis of the mediating role of life satisfaction in the relationship between automatic thoughts and depression.

4. Discussion

In this study, the relationships between depression, negative automatic thoughts, life satisfaction that is a part of subjective well-being and attributions used by people while interpreting physical symptoms and life events were examined in a sample of teacher candidates. First, pre-analysis was conducted to determine whether there were gender differences in DS, ATS, SIQ subscales scores and LSS scores. As a result of the analysis, it is found that female teacher candidates' SIQ NS and P subscale scores and LSS scores were higher compared to males (**Table 1**). In addition, SIQ NS subscale scores of teacher candidates who encountered an event causing stress during the past 3 months were higher than the scores of others (see **Table 1**). Depression scores of young adults did not show difference according to gender and whether they encountered an event-causing stress during the past 3 months or not. In literature regarding depression, the studies on gender differences put forward different results. Some studies found that depression levels of males were higher than the females (For example, see [65]); some found that depression levels of females were higher than the males (For example, see [66]) and some found that gender did not create a difference on the depression level (for example, see [67–69]). In literature examining the relationship between stressful life events and depression, it is stated that life events are both stressful and an important risk factor when they accumulate [46, 70]. In his study, independent from personality traits and type of event, Kabakçı [71] found that groups with medium or high-level depression had encountered an event causing high-level stress during the past 6 months compared to the group that did not show depressive symptoms. Similarly, it was found significant relationships between depression and daily social and academic problems. However, it is emphasized that not everybody experiencing stressful life events show depressive symptoms. What causes depression is not having enough strength and ability to cope with these events [47].

In correlation analysis, positive correlation between teacher candidates' DS scores and ATS, SIQ, NS, *P*, S and N subscale scores and negative correlation between their DS scores and LSS scores were found (see **Table 2**). Another finding was that five variables (ATS, LSS, SIQ NS, P and N subscales) are significant predictors in explaining the depression level of young adults (see **Table 3**). Together, these five variables explain 52% of the young adults' depression. The biggest contribution to the prediction of depression scores of young adults came from automatic thoughts with 42%. This finding shows similarity to the study findings stating a relationship between automatic thoughts and depression [67, 72–76]. Automatic thoughts have also been identified as predictors of negative mood states [77] and negative emotions [78]. Automatic thoughts are defined as repeated negative or positive automatic self-statements that an individual repeats to him/herself in certain situations. People generally accept these thoughts as correct without thinking about them critically [79]. How the individual perceives negatively himself, his life experiences and his future is named as "negative trilogy" by Beck and it explains almost all symptoms of depression [80]. A person who is in depression perceives himself as worthless, inefficient, morally handicapped and he blames himself for his negative experiences and he thinks that others do not like him. Furthermore, he thinks that too many things were demanded from him and that the world is full of insurmountable obstacles. He perceives the future as dark, prone to failure and as a hopeless situation [80].

http://dx.doi.org/10.5772/66622

Life satisfaction comes second in the prediction of young adults' depression scores. According to this finding, life satisfaction is a negative predictor of depression. In the literature, there are studies showing negative relationship between depression and life satisfaction [40, 81–85]. Life satisfaction is closely related to psychological health. It was found that people with general anxiety disorder and major depression have lower life satisfaction scores than the general population [83]. The people who have high life satisfaction are those who assess their life events and life circumstances in a positive way. Depression includes affects like pessimism, sadness, hopelessness and loneliness [86]. In this context, life satisfaction being negative predictor of depression is an expected result. The type of symptom attribution has the least contribution to the prediction of depression scores of young adults. The results of analysis indicate that number of symptoms, psychologizing and normalizing were significant predictors in explaining the depression level of young adults. In their study, where they examined the relationship between symptom attribution type and physical symptoms of depression, Güleç et al. [87] found a low relationship between mental attributions of people with depression and depression values. As a result, in their study, they found that the depressive group did not have a tendency to interpret their symptoms using any of the attribution types [87]. The mediator role of life satisfaction on the relation between automatic thoughts and depression especially was the major question of this study. It was found that LSS partially mediated the relationship between ATS and DS for the young adults (see **Table 4**). In other words, negative automatic thoughts of young adults cause them to negatively assess their quality of life and this situation leads to an increase in the depression level. Based on this study, it can be argued for interactions between automatic thoughts, depression and life satisfaction.

In this study, negative automatic thoughts, life satisfaction, stressful life events and symptom attribution types were discussed as predictors of depression. There can be variables (self-esteem, loneliness, resilience, neuroticism, social support, coping strategies etc..) other than this study's variables in explaining depression among young adults. One of the limitations of the study is that the study group is composed of teacher candidates between the ages of 21 and 29 who were not diagnosed with depression. In the future, a clearer picture of the current situation can be drawn by working on a model examining the aforementioned variables and sample group that was diagnosed with depression. Another limitation is that data is based on teacher candidates' self-report. Responses provided by choosing items from the scale may not truly represent real behaviors of the teacher candidates. Therefore, results should be interpreted within the limitations of the scales.

5. Conclusion

Conducted with young adults, this study's findings reveal that negative automatic thoughts, life satisfaction and symptom attribution type (a number of symptoms, psychologizing and normalizing) are significant predictors in explaining depression levels of young adults. In addition, life satisfaction is a partial mediator in the relationship between negative automatic thoughts and depression. As a result negative automatic thoughts of young adults cause them to negatively assess their quality of life and this situation leads to an increase in the depression level.

Author details

Yasemin Yavuzer[1]* and Zeynep Karataş[2]

*Address all correspondence to: yyavuzer@hotmail.com

1 Faculty of Education Department of Guidance and Counselling, Ömer Halisdemir University, Nigde, Turkey

2 Faculty of Education Department of Guidance and Counselling, Mehmet Akif Ersoy University, Burdur, Turkey

References

[1] WHO (2016). Programme on mental health. Measuring quality of life. Retrieved 3 September 2016 from http://www.who.int/mental_health/media/68.pdf.

[2] Akdeniz, C. & Aydemir, Ö. (1999). Adaptatıon and relıabılıty analysıs of health measurement questıonnaıre. Bull.Clin.Psychopharmacol., 9(2), 104–108.

[3] Cicchett, D. & Toth, S. (1998). The development of depression in children and adolescents. American Psychologist, 53, 221–241.

[4] Steinberg, L. (2002). Adolescence. (Sixth Edition). Boston: McGraw-Hill, pp. 444–452.

[5] Davison, G.C. & Neale, J.M. (2004). Abnormal Psychology. (Trans. Ed. İhsan Dağ). Ankara: Turkish Psychologists Association Publications.

[6] Gökçakan, Z. & Gökçakan, N. (2005). Cognitive therapy on depression. Mersin University Journal of the Faculty of Education, 1(1), 91–101.

[7] Erdoğan, G. (2006). The effects of creatıve drama on the self-concept and depressıve symptoms of 8th grade (ages 14–15) students wıth depressıve symptoms. Master's thesis, Gazi University, Ankara, Turkey.

[8] Shapiro, P.G. (1997). Childhood and first youth depression. (Translate. Meral Kesim). İstanbul: Papirüs.

[9] Kesler, R.C., Berglund, P., Demler, O, Jin, R., Karetz, D., Merikangas, K.R. Rush, A.J., Walters, E.E. & Wang, P.S. (2003). The epidemiology of major depressive disorder. Results from the Nationality Comorbitity Survey Replication (NCS-R). Journal of the American Medical Association, 289(23), 3095–3105.

[10] Küçükkendirci, H. (2000). The relationship between socio demographic characteristic and the depression scan results with children depression inventory in the students primary school (Part two). Doctoral dissertation, Selçuk University, Konya, Turkey.

[11] Kaya, B. (2007). Depression: Socio-economic and cultural perspectives. Journal of Clinical Psychiatry, 10(6), 11–20.

[12] Costello, E.J., Costello, A.J., Edelbrock, C., Burns, B.J., Dulcan, M.K., Brent, D.A. & Janiszewski, S. (1988). Psychiatric disorders in pediatric primary care: Prevalence and risk factors. Archives of General Psychiatry, 45, 1107–1116.

[13] Parker, G., Cheah, Y.C. & Roy, K. (2001). Do the Chinese somatize depression? A cross cultural study. Social Psychiatry and Psychiatric Epidemiology, 36(6), 287–293.

[14] Angold, A., Erkanli, A., Farmer, E., Fairbank, J.A., Burns, B.J., Keeler, G. & Costello, E.J. (2002). Psychiatric disorder impairment and service use in rural African and white youth. Archives of General Psychiatry, 59, 893–901.

[15] Ebert, D. & Martus, P. (1994) Somatization as a core symptom of melancolic type depression. Evidence from a cross-cultural study. Journal of Affect Disorder, 32, 253–256.

[16] Uluşahin, A., Başoğlu, M. & Paykel, E.S. (1994). A cross cultural comparative study of depressive symptoms in British and Turkish clinical samples. Social Psychiatry and Psychiatric Epidemiology, 29(1), 31–39.

[17] Akbıyık, İ.D., Mendel, E.G., Önder, E.M. & Cording, C. (1999). The effects of being an "immigrant" on the symptoms of depression of the Turkish people living in Germany. Journal of Crisis, 7(2), 25–29.

[18] Anderson, C.A. (1999). Attributional style, depression and loneliness: a cross-cultural comparison of American and Chinese students. PSBP, 25(4), 482–499.

[19] Twenge, J.M. & Nolen-Hoeksema, S. (2002). Age, gender, race, socioeconomic status and birth cohort differences on the Children's Depression Inventory: A meta-analysis. Journal of Abnormal Psychology, 111(4), 578–588.

[20] Lee, E.E. & Farran, C.J. (2004). Depression among Korean, Korean American and Caucasian American family caregivers. Journal of Transcultural Nursing, 15(1), 18–25.

[21] Lawrence, V., Murray, J., Banerjee, S., Turner, S., Sangha, K., Byng, R., Bhugra, D., Huxley, P., Tylee, A. & Macdonald, A. (2005). Concepts and causation of depression: a cross-cultural study of the beliefs of older adults. The Gerontologist, 46(1), 23–32.

[22] Colla, J., Buka, S., Harrington, D. & Murphy, J.M. (2006). Depression and modernization: a cross-cultural study of women. Social Psychiatry and Psychiatric Epidemiology, 41(4), 271–279.

[23] Khawaia, N.G., Santos, ML, R.R., Habibi, M. & Smith, R. (2011). University students' depression: a cross-cultural investigation. Higher Education Research and Development, 32(3), 392–406.

[24] Karataş, Z. & Tremblay, R.E. (2015). Analyzing the levels of depressive symptoms among secondary school students in Canada and Turkey. Cypriot Journal of Educational Sciences, 10(3), 245–256.

[25] Türkçapar, M.H., Sungur, M.Z. & Akdemir, A. (1994). Cognitive therapies in children and adolescents. Turkish Journal of Child and Adolescent Mental Health, 2(2), 93–100.

[26] Beck, A.T. (1976). Cognitive therapy and the emotional disorders. New York: International University Press.

[27] Bozkurt, N. (1998). The relationship between depression, automatic thoughts and school achievements in high school students. Doctoral dissertation, Dokuz Eylül University, İzmir, Turkey.

[28] Heffron, K. & Boniwell, I. (2014). Positive psychology (Trans. Ed. T. Doğan). Ankara: Nobel.

[29] Diener, E. (1984). Subjective well being. Psychological Bulletin, 95(3), 542–575.

[30] Akın, A. (2013). Subjective well-being. In Current psychological concepts I, Positive psychology (Ed. A. Akın). Sakarya: Sakarya University Educational Sciences Institute Publications.

[31] Tuzgöl Dost, M. (2005). Mental health and subjective well-being. Eurasian Journal of Educational Research, 20, 223–231.

[32] Joshanloo, M. (2013). The influence of fear of happiness beliefs on responses to the satisfaction with life scale. Personality and Individual Differences, 54, 647–651.

[33] McDowell, I. (2010). Measures of self-perceived well-being. Journal of Psychosomatic, 69, 69–76.

[34] Joshi, U. (2010). Subjective well-being by gender. Journal of Economics and Behavioral Studies, 1(1), 20–26.

[35] Diener, E., Suh, E.M, Lucas, R.E., & Smith, H.L (1999). Subjective well-being: three decades of progress. Psychological Bulletin, 125(2), 276–302.

[36] Pavot,W. & Diener, E. (1993). The affective and cognitive context of self reported measures of subjective well-being. Social Indicators Research, 28, 1–20.

[37] Deniz, M.E. (2006). The relationships among coping with stress, life satisfaction, decision making styles and decision self-esteem: An investigation with Turkish University Students. Social Behaviour and Personality, 34(9), 1161–1170.

[38] Diener, E., Emmons, R.A., Larsen, R.J., & Griffin, S. (1985). The satisfaction with life scale. Journal of Personality Assessment, 49, 71–75.

[39] Diener, E. & Lucas, R.E. (1999). Subjective well-being: three decades of progress. Psychological Bulletin, 125 (2), 276–303.

[40] Diener, E. & Ryan, K. (2009). Subjective well-being: a general overview. South African Journal of Psychology, 39, 391–406.

[41] Bailey, R.C., & Miller, C. (1998). Life satisfaction and life demands in college students. Social Behavior and Personality, 26(1), 51–56.

[42] Çeçen, A.R. (2007). The Turkish version of the social and emotional loneliness scale for adults (SELSA-S): initial development and validation. Social Behaviour and Personality, 35(6), 717–734.

[43] Yetim, Ü. (2003) The impacts of individualism/collectivism, selfesteem and feeling of mastery on life satisfaction among the Turkish university students and academicians. Social Indicators Research, 61, 297–317.

[44] Gündoğar, D., Sallan Gül, S., Uskun, E., Demirci, S. & Keçeci, D. (2007). Investigation of the predictors of life satisfaction in university students. Journal of Clinical Psychiatry, 10, 14–27.

[45] Doğan, T. (2006). The ınvestıgatıon of the wellness of unıversıty students. H.U. Journal of Education, 30, 120–129.

[46] Eskin, M., Akoğlu, A. & Uygur, B. (2006). Traumatic life events and problem solving skills in psychiatric outpatients: Relationships with suicidal behavior, Turkish Journal of Psychiatry, 17(4), 266–275.

[47] Josepho, S.A., Plutchik, R. (1994). Stress, coping and suicide risk in psychiatric inpatients. Suicide and Life-Threatening Behavior, 24, 48–57.

[48] Duman, O.Y. Usubutun, S. & Göka, E. (2004). Validity and reliability of the Turkish form of symptom ınterpretation questionnaire. Turkish Journal of Psychiatry, 15, 26–40.

[49] Robbins, J.M. & Kirmayer, L.J. (1991). Attributions of common somatic symptoms. Psychological Medicine, 21, 1029–1045.

[50] Özen, E.M., Serhadlı, Z.N.A., Türkcan, A.S. & Ülker, G.E. (2010). Somatization in depression and anxiety disorders. The Journal of Psychiatry and Neurological Sciences, 23(1), 60–65.

[51] Lipowski ZJ. (1990). Somatization and depression. Psychosomatics, 31, 13–21.

[52] Eryılmaz, A. & Ercan, L. (2010). Initiaing romantic ıntimacy at emerging adulthood: Is it intimacy or isolation? Journal of Turkish Psychological Counseling and Guidance, 4(34), 119–127.

[53] Evans, S.W (1999) Mental health services in schools: Utilization, effectiveness and consent. Clininical Psychology Review, 19(2),165–178.

[54] Kaya, M., Genç, M., Kaya, B. & Pehlivan, E. (2007). Prevalence of depressive symptoms, ways of coping, and related factors among medical school and health services higher education students. Turkish Journal of Psychiatry, 18(2), 137–146.

[55] Hisli, N. (1988). A study on the validity of the Beck depression inventory. Journal of Psychology, 6, 118–126.

[56] Köker, S. (1991). Comparison of life satisfaction levels of normal and troubled adolescents. Master's thesis, Ankara University, Ankara, Turkey.

[57] Yetim, Ü. (1993). Life satisfaction: A study based on the organization of personal projects. Social Indicators Research, 29, 277–289.

[58] Hollon, S.D. & Kendall, P.C. (1980). Cognitive self-statements in depression: Development of an automatic thoughts questionnaire. Cognitive Therapy and Research, 4(4), 383–395.

[59] Şahin, N.H. & Şahin, N. (1992). Reliability and validity of the Turkish version of the automatic thoughts questionnaire. Journal of Clinical Psychology, 48,51–57.

[60] Savaşır, I. & Şahin, N.H. (1997). Evaluation in cognitive behavioral therapies: Frequently used scales. Ankara: Turkish Psychologists Association Publications, pp. 29–30.

[61] Karaatli, M. (2006). Regulation and representation of the data: In Kalaycioglu S (editor). SPSS Applied Multivariate Statistical Techniques. Second Edition, Ankara: Asil Publication Distribution, pp. 3–47. (Turkish)

[62] Tabachnick, B.G., & Fidell, L.S. (2001). Using multivariate statistics. Fourth Edition. Boston, MA: Allyn and Bacon.

[63] Stevens, J.P. (2002). Applied multivariate statistics for the social sciences. Fourth Edition. Mahwah, New Jersey: Lawrence Erlbaum Associates, Publishers.

[64] Baron, R.M., & Kenny, D.A. (1986). The moderator-mediator variable distinction in social psychological research: Conceptual, strategic and statistical considerations. Journal of Personality and Social Psychology, 51(6), 1173–1182.

[65] Tuzcuoğlu, S. & Korkmaz, B. (2001). Investigating the levels of submissive behavior and depression among psychological counseling and guidance university students. M.Ü. Atatürk Journal of Education Faculty Educational Sciences, 14, 135–152.

[66] Yücel, B. Kara, K., Özyalçın, S., Alçalar, N., Özdemir, Ö. & Yücel, A. (2002). Depression, automatic thoughts, alexithymia and assertiveness in patients with tension-type headache. Headache, 42, 194–199.

[67] Aysan, F. & Bozkurt, N. (2000). The relationships beıween students' coping strategies and their negative automatic thoughts and depression levels. Journal of Marmara University Educational Sciences, 12, 25–38.

[68] Donnelly, R., Renk, K., Sims, V.K. & McGuire, J. (2011). The relationship between parents' and children's automatic thoughts in a college student sample. Child Psychiatry and Human Development, 42, 197–218.

[69] Ören, N. & Gençdoğan, B. (2007). The analysıs of the depressıon levels of the lycee students accordıng to some varıables. Kastamonu Education Journal, 15(1), 85–92.

[70] Algül, A., Özşahin, A., Ateş, M.A., Başoğlu, C., Semiz, Ü.B., Ebrinç, S., Doruk, A. Perdeci, Z. & Çetim, M. (2009). The relationship between the menopausal depression and previous depressive episode, and family history of depression, and life events. Bulletin of Clinical Psychopharmacology, 19(1), 247–249.

[71] Kabakçı, E. (2001). Sociotropic/autonomic personality characteristics, life events and depressive symptoms among university students. Turkish Journal of Psychiatry, 12(4), 273–282.

[72] Calvete, E. & Connor-Smith, J.K. (2005). Automatic thoughts and psychological symptoms: A cross-cultural comparison of American and Spanish students. Cognitive Therapy and Research, 29(2), 201–17.

[73] Clarke, D. & Goosen, T. (2009). The mediating effects of coping strategies in the relationship between automatic negative thoughts and depression in a clinical sample of diabetes patients. Personality and Individual Differences, 46, 460–464.

http://dx.doi.org/10.5772/66622

[74] Hjemdal, O., Stiles, T. & Wells, A. (2013). Automatic thoughts and meta-cognition as predictors of depressive or anxious symptoms: A prospective study of two trajectories. Scandinavian Journal of Psychology, 54, 59–65.

[75] Kercher, A.J., Rapee, R.M. & Schniering, C.A. (2009). Neuroticism, life events and negative thoughts in the development of depression in adolescent girls. Journal of Abnormal Child Psychology, 37, 903–915.

[76] Vatanasin, D., Thapinta, D., Thompson, E.A. & Thungjaroenkul, P. (2012). Testing a model of depression among thai adolescents. Journal of Child and Adolescent Psychiatric Nursing, 25, 195–206.

[77] McHugh, K. & Wierzbicki, M. (1998). Prediction of responses to cognitive and behavioral mood inductions. Journal of Psychology, 132, 33–41.

[78] Schniering, C.A. & Rapee, R.M. (2004). The relationship between automatic thoughts and negative emotions in children and adolescents: A test of the cognitive content-specificity hypothesis. Journal of Abnormal Psychology, 113(3), 464–70.

[79] Beck, J.S. (2001). Cognitive Therapy: Basic Principles and Beyond. (Translate. N Hisli Şahin), (Trans. Ed. F Balkaya, A İlden Koçkar), Ankara: Turkish Psychologists Association Publications.

[80] Savaşır, I. & Yıldız, S. (1996). Cognitive-behavioral treatment of depression. In Savaşır I, Boyacıoğlu G, Kabakçı E (editors). Cognitive-Behavioral Therapies. Ankara: Turkish Psychologists Association Publications, pp. 17–49.

[81] Karakuş, M. & Çankaya, İ.H. (2012). Examining a model related to mobbing incurred by teachers. H.U. Journal of Education, 42, 225–237.

[82] Serin, N.B., Serin, O. & Özbaş, L.F. (2010). Predicting university students' life satisfaction by their anxiety and depression level. Procedia Social and Behavioral Sciences, 9, 579–582.

[83] Stein, M.B. & Heimberg, R.G. (2004).Well-being and life satisfaction in generalized anxiety disorder: Comparison to major depressive disorder in a community sample. Journal of Affective Disorders, 79, 161–166.

[84] Yavuzer, Y. & Çivilidag, A. (2014). Mediator role of depression on the relationship between mobbing and life satisfaction of health professionals. The Journal of Psychiatry and Neurological Sciences, 27(2), 115–125.

[85] Yıldırım, A. & Hacıhasanoğlu, R. (2011). Quality of life and effective variables among health care professionals. Journal of Psychiatric Nursing, 2, 61–68.

[86] Köknel, Ö. (2005). Depression, mental depression. Istanbul: Golden Books Publishing.

[87] Güleç, H., Sayar, K. & Özkorumak, E. (2005). Somatic symptoms of Depression. Turkish Journal of Psychiatry, 16(2), 90–96.

Chapter 6

Body-Mind Connectedness: Integrative Body-Mind-Spirit Group Work for Depressed Persons with Salient Somatic Disturbances

Sylvia Hong Yao, Jane Xiao-Wen Ji,
Celia Hoi Yan Chan and Cecilia Lai Wan Chan

Additional information is available at the end of the chapter

http://dx.doi.org/10.5772/66960

Abstract

Globally, depression frequently comorbid with a variety of physical illnesses, which exert substantial mental and somatic distresses on patients. Sleep disturbance is one of the common conditions reported by individuals with either, mental or physical illnesses. Complex interaction among depression, sleep and physical illnesses highlighted the essential mind-body connection in the planning of integrative care and other clinical services. A number of eastern mind-body practices, such as Qigong, acupuncture and meditation, have been frequently studied indicating the efficacy of mind-body connection in complementary therapies. This chapter will introduce the integrative body-mind-spirit (I-BMS) group work, which has been found effective in addressing comorbid depressed mood and somatic afflictions, especially sleep disturbances among Hong Kong Chinese adults.

Keywords: depression, somatic symptoms, sleep disturbances, mind-body connection, integrative body-mind-spirit (I-BMS)

1. Introduction

Depression is one of the most common mental illnesses across the world. Individuals with depression may also present a number of bodily symptoms, such as insomnia, pain, fatigue, vitality loss as well as unpleasant sensations of loss of appetite, weight, bodily and emotional tension or heaviness [1]. There are gender differences in the expression of somatic symptoms among depressive patients. Depressed women tended to show decreased eating/sleeping symptoms and reduced or increased appetite/weight and hypersomnia; however, men with depression can express melancholic retardation and agitated depression based on psychomotor activities [2].

Depression, together with somatic disturbances, is largely responsible for psychosocial impediments of clinical patients. Somatic disturbances and depressive mood seem to be reciprocally correlated. The somatic symptoms, such as sleep disturbance, are certainly associated with onset and development of depression [3]. Moreover, depression has been found to increase the risk development and severity of chronic illness in longitudinal studies [4]. In both literature and practice, the interplay between depression and somatic syndromes is not well understood. Hence, more works are required to better understand how this close association between depression and somatic/physical distresses can further inform existing models of depression.

A great deal of studies has consistently found that insomnia can predict the onset of depression and might perpetuate the residual depression symptoms among patients in remission [5]. Some studies indicated a bidirectional relation between insomnia and depression [5]. Some other studies only found a unidirectional relationship between sleep problems at baseline and incident of depression later, but not vice versa [6]. Buysse and associates conducted a 20-year study to understand comorbidity of insomnia and depression, and found that either insomnia occurred with or without depression, it is highly stable over time if not treated [7]. More importantly, it is the comorbid syndrome rather than standalone insomnia or depression tended to longitudinally relate to future diagnosis. Thus, it seems essential to consider these two conditions under an integrative framework.

With a holistic perspective, integrative body-mind-spirit model is an approach derived from Eastern philosophies and therapeutic techniques to create positive and transformative changes in individuals and families [8]. Randomized clinical trials have been conducted to examine the effectiveness of this approach in treatments of depression, anxiety, posttraumatic stress disorders, prolonged grief and so forth [9–11]. The IBMS intervention was usually delivered in the group modality on a weekly basis. In a mixed study of effectiveness of I-BMS for clinical depression, researchers delivered thematic psycho-education and breathing exercises, and guided imaginary hand massage, one-second techniques, etc., for patients with clinical diagnosis of depression [12]. After intervention, participants were able to accept their depression and the physical, emotional and spiritual changes caused by depression, more importantly, learn to appreciate and practice body-mind connection in therapeutic context and in their daily routines. Similar designs have found positive outcomes of I-BMS across different cultural contexts [13].

This chapter will introduce the significance of the body-mind connectedness in the health-promoting practices for patients with depressive symptoms. Furthermore, this chapter will also present the integrative body-mind-spirit model and its effectiveness in reducing the depressive symptoms and enhancing the overall quality of life for people with comorbid depressive symptoms and sleep problems.

2. Behavioral medicine for depression: mind-body bridging

A reciprocal relationship between mental and physical health highlighted the significant role of mind-body connection in health service. An online survey on depressed patients and professionals even suggested that discussing mind-body connection could help to improve diagnosis and management of depression [14]. Lots of mind-body techniques had been adopted to promote mental and physical health, including physical exercises, Qigong, yoga, acupuncture and mindful meditation.

a) Physical exercises

Regular physical activities can arguably benefit both physical and mental health as showed by studies in medicine and social sciences. Exercises have been viewed as an imperative dimension on lifestyle modifications in prevention, management and recovery of chronic illness, including depression [15]. In fact, physical exercises may be more applicable for those with mild and moderate depression who are more motivated and capable to engage in physical activities than those under severe conditions [16]. According to a meta-analysis, physical exercises can significantly reduce depression symptoms and improve the treatment responses. However, the efficacy of physical exercises in the treatment of depression was influenced by age and baseline depression severity [17].

b) Exercise Qigong

Qigong is an ancient Chinese mind-body practice, originated from ancient thoughts of inner healing and informed traditional Chinese medicine practices. It is designed to cultivate life force (*Qi*), a vital energy that sustains holistic well-being. Nowadays, Qigong has developed into different schools, but most forms of exercise Qigong comprise a series of orchestrated practices including body postures such as standing or sitting, the performance of a range of simple movements, breathing techniques and meditation to attain a deeply focused state of easiness that were addressed along the history. Besides health maintenance, exercise Qigong has been found effective in fostering patients' recovery from cancer and noncancer diseases. A randomized trial control study found that medical exercise Qigong could improve cancer patient's overall quality of life and mood status and simultaneously reduced side effects of cancer treatments [18]. Exercise Qigong has also been applied to improve neurologic, immune and respiratory functions, which possibly associated with better health and mental health [19, 20]. In terms of depression, the effectiveness of exercise Qigong in treatment of depression has found to be positive in Chinese context [21].

c) Acupuncture

Acupuncture is the insertion and stimulation of needles at specific points on the body to relieve pain and facilitate restoration of health. It is a traditional medicine intervention practiced in China and other Asian countries for thousands of years. Randomized trial studies have demonstrated that acupuncture is beneficial to reducing symptoms of depression [22], posttraumatic stress disorders [23], postpartum stresses [24] as well as other psychosocial-emotional problems. However, the placebo of acupuncture required further researches as indicated by a randomized study that showed that placebo acupuncture significantly predicted higher overall pregnancy rate through reducing stress and anxiety levels in comparison with real acupuncture [25].

d) Mindful meditation

Mindful meditation is derived from Buddhist practices. Comparing to "pure" meditation, the mindfulness-centered program has its most powerful effect on reducing stress and improving psychological health [26]. Thus, mindful meditation is a research-based form of meditation designed to achieve moment-to-moment attentions to flow of experiences, a modern psychological term defined as "the awareness that emerges through paying attention on purpose, in the present moment, and nonjudgmentally to the unfolding of experience moment by moment" [27]. The main goal of mindful meditation is to develop skills of paying attention to our inner and outer experiences with acceptance, patience and self-compassion. As a complementary approach, mindful-based stress reduction and mindful-based cognitive therapy had demonstrated antidepressant and antianxiety effects among patients with chronic illnesses, patients with mental disorders as well as healthy populations [28]. In particular, self-compassion is an important therapeutic element in mindful-based intervention and can predict improved emotional well-being of practitioners over a long term [29].

3. I-BMS practice: valuing and integrating the body, mind and spiritual connection

The integrative body-mind-spirit (I-BMS) model is an integrative approach derived from traditional Chinese medicine, Confucianism and Daoism [30]. Core beliefs of the I-BMS model include (a) the interconnectedness of body, mind and soul (spirit), (b) the importance of spirituality as a domain of human existence, (c) the need to reach beyond symptom reduction to attain growth and transformative changes and (d) the multiple goals of healing, empowerment, love and forgiveness as well as capacity building [31]. Besides Eastern philosophical teachings, integrative body-mind-spirit model is inspired to derive wisdom from Western medicine, counseling and psychotherapy.

With a holistic perspective, I-BMS acknowledged and utilized the power of the body, mind, spirit and the universe. By so doing, one can reach beyond physical and psychological symptoms reduction to the attainment of emotional and spiritual transformation. Therefore, positive and transformative changes could happen in the physical, cognition, emotional and social domains, core values and meanings, as well as the religious connection with the higher being and their inner self. Core principles of mind-body medicine have been applied in the I-BMS model to promote responsible health care.

The core principles of mind-body medicine [32]

- Mind-body medicine is a way of perceiving and practicing medicine that mirrors and integrates every facet of life.
- Mind-body medicine weaves together the central components that contribute to an individual's experience, and in so doing honors that weaving as a sum greater than its individual parts.
- The practice of mind-body medicine makes it incumbent upon physicians to develop life skills so as to promote understanding, respect and value for others.
- Mind-body medicine emphasizes the concept of healing as much as it does curing.

Integrative body-mind-spirit model conceived depression as a manifestation of body-mind-spirit unbalance, and thus, the ultimate therapeutic goal is not only to enhance moods of depressed patients, but also to facilitate participants to realize, define and reconstruct unbalanced experiences by coordinating bodily, emotional and spiritual domains [33]. In addition to counseling, indigenous mind-body techniques, including relaxation techniques, grass roots yoga, breathing exercises, Qigong, Tai chi exercises and body scan, were used to treat patients with depressed mood and improve the psychosocial well-being of cancer patients, bereaved persons, divorced individuals and women with infertility using the I-BMS model [9–11]. These mind-body techniques have been proven beneficial in reducing depression and anxiety symptoms among mental illness patients [34].

In order to reduce depressive symptoms and improve holistic well-being for people with sleep problems, a randomized, waiting list control trial has been conducted during 2013–2015. A total of 1002 adults with self-reporting sleep problems from community show their participatory intentions for I-BMS intervention. All interested participants are invited complete online questionnaires, consisting of Center for Epidemiologic Studies Depression Scale (CESD), Somatic Symptom Index (SSI), Pittsburgh Sleep Quality Index (PSQI) and other psychosocial measures. Based on calculated sample size, this study randomly selected 200 individuals who reported mild-to-moderate depression ($34 \geq CESD \geq 10$) and sleep disturbances with self-reported insomnia (PSQI >5) based on a computer-generated number list. Followed by random control trial protocol, 185 eligible participants were randomly selected assigned into either an I-BMS intervention group ($n = 92$) or a waiting list control group ($n = 93$), except 15 participants without valid consent form in the pool. The I-BMS group intervention is delivered on weekly base with eight sessions, themed by culturally specific mind-body exercise, mindful meditation, self-reflection and group sharing [35, 36]. This I-BMS intervention for individuals with comorbid depressive and sleep disturbances integrated the mind-body techniques:

- Acupressure
- Breathing meditation
- Body scans
- Qigong exercises
- Hand massage exercises
- Loving-kindness meditation
- Guided imaginary
- Gratitude, forgiveness and appreciation exercises
- Group discussions

4. Effectiveness of I-BMS group intervention for current sleep and mood disturbances

It is found that the I-BMS intervention can effectively improve participants' sleep quality and depressive mood immediately after treatment, and the effect was maintained at the 3-month follow-up with large within-group effect size (ES: 0.74–1.08). The remission rate of clinically significant depressive symptoms (CESD ≥ 16) was significantly greater in the I-BMS group than that of the control group at both posttreatment and follow-up. Specifically, half of individuals with significant depressive symptoms had a remission after I-BMS treatment in comparison with only less than quarter remission in WLC group. More importantly, the I-BMS also successfully reduces expression of inflammatory cytokines, interleukin 6, in comparison with control groups [37]. These findings lend further support for study of mind-body connection in depressive disorders, and the holistic effects yield of I-BMS group intervention on human subjects. Moreover, a bi-directional relation was found between change in sleep quality and improvement in depressive mood at the 3-month follow-up that highlighted the interactions between the mind and the body in the context of a holistic intervention [38, 39]. In addition to sleep disturbances, many other somatic distresses are also found decreased following the I-BMS treatment by fixed-effect linear model. Study flow and detailed information on participants can be found in aforementioned articles. In fact, there are significant time × group interaction effects on somatic subscale of somatic symptom inventory (SSI) [$F(2, 411) = 4.68$, $p = 0.01$)], bodily irritability measured by holistic well-being scale [$F(2, 411)$ 3.12, $p = 0.045$)] and general vitality, also measured by holistic well-being scale [$F(2, 411)$ 10.24, $p < 0.001$)] favoring I-BMS group. Forward analysis would be required to understand the associations between changes in mood and that in somatic disturbances other than sleep, such as fatigue, headache and lack of vitality.

5. Conclusion

Somatic symptoms play a vital role in diagnosis, prevention and management of depression, either comorbid with or without other medical conditions. The physical and mental needs of depressive individuals required the catered psychosocial supports and interventions emphasizing on the body-mind connection. In this chapter, we try to examine and explain the values of Integrative body-mind-spirit model in reducing the comorbid depressive and somatic symptoms. After I-BMS intervention conducted in Hong Kong, a randomized control trial study found the positive changes in sleep quality, immediate and long-term depressive mood. Moreover, the I-BMS also successfully reduces expression of inflammatory cytokines, interleukin 6, in comparison with control groups. The improvement in psychical biomarkers and psychometric index may suggest the effectiveness of body-mind techniques conducted in I-BMS. All these exciting findings emphasize on promoting mind-body connection in the development of I-BMS and other psychosocial caring models for individuals with depression, especially comorbid with varied medical conditions. Forward analysis

http://dx.doi.org/10.5772/66960

would be encouraged to understand the associations between changes in mood and that in somatic disturbances other than sleep, such as fatigue, headache and lack of vitality. In practice, more integrative and innovative therapeutic modalities helping bridging mind-body are warranted to optimize treatments for individuals with depressive symptoms and other medical conditions.

Author details

Sylvia Hong Yao[1], Jane Xiao-Wen Ji[1], Celia Hoi Yan Chan[1, 2]* and Cecilia Lai Wan Chan[1, 2]

*Address all correspondence to: chancelia@hku.hk

1 Department of Social Work and Social Administration, The University of Hong Kong, Hong Kong SAR, China

2 Centre on Behavioral Health, The University of Hong Kong, Hong Kong SAR, China

References

[1] Aktas, A., Walsh, D., Hauser, K., & Rybicki, L. (2016). Should we cluster patients or symptoms? The myth of symptom clusters based on 'depression, insomnia, pain' and 'depression, fatigue, pain'. BMJ Supportive & Palliative Care, 6(2), 210–218.

[2] Alexandrino-Silva, C., Wang, Y. P., Viana, M. C., Bulhões, R. S., Martins, S. S., & Andrade, L. H. (2013). Gender differences in symptomatic profiles of depression: results from the Sao Paulo Megacity Mental Health Survey. Journal of Affective Disorders, 147(1), 355–364.

[3] Tylee, A., & Gandhi, P. (2005). The importance of somatic symptoms in depression in primary care. Primary Care Companion to The Journal of Clinical Psychiatry, 7(4), 167–76.

[4] Nicholson, A., Kuper, H., & Hemingway, H. (2006). Depression as an aetiologic and prognostic factor in coronary heart disease: a meta-analysis of 6362 events among 146 538 participants in 54 observational studies. European Heart Journal, 27:2763–2774.

[5] Baglioni, C., Spiegelhalder, K., Lombardo, C., & Riemann, D. (2010). Sleep and emotions: a focus on insomnia. Sleep Medicine Reviews, 14(4), 227–238.

[6] Johnson, E. O., Roth, T., & Breslau, N. (2006). The association of insomnia with anxiety disorders and depression: exploration of the direction of risk. Journal of Psychiatric Research, 40(8), 700–708.

[7] Buysse, D. J., Angst, J., Gamma, A., Ajdacic, V., Eich, D., & Rossler, W. (2008). Prevalence, course, and comorbidity of insomnia and depression in young adults. Sleep-New York then Westchester, 31(4), 473.

[8] Lee, M. Y., Ng, S. M., Leung, P. P. Y., & Chan, C. L. W. (2009). Integrative body-mind-spirit social work: An empirically based approach to assessment and treatment. New York: Oxford Univeristy Press.

[9] Chan, C. L., Chan, Y., & Lou, V. W. (2002). Evaluating an empowerment group for divorced Chinese women in Hong Kong. Research on Social Work Practice, 12(4), 558–569.

[10] Chan, C. L. W. (2001). An Eastern body–mind–spirit approach: a training manual with one-second techniques. Hong Kong: Department of Social work and Social Administration, The University of Hong Kong. Resource Paper Series No. 43.

[11] Leung, P. P. Y. (1997). Stress management for cancer patients: a psycho-educational-support group. In C. L. W. Chan & N. Rhind (Eds.), Social work intervention in health care: The Hong Kong scene (pp. 85–103). Hong Kong: Hong Kong University Press.

[12] Lee, M. Y., Ng, S. M., Leung, P. P. Y., & Chan, C. L. W. (2009). Integrative body-mind-spirit social work: an empirically based approach to assessment and treatment. New York: Oxford Univeristy Press.

[13] Sreevani, R., Reddemma, K., Chan, C. L., Leung, P. P., Wong, V., & Chan, C. H. (2013). Effectiveness of integrated body-mind-spirit group intervention on the well-being of Indian patients with depression: a pilot study. Journal of Nursing Research, 21(3), 179–186. doi: 10.1097/jnr.0b013e3182a0b041

[14] Cited from Luczaj S. (2007). http://counsellingresource.com/features/2007/10/23/depression-mind-body/

[15] Martinsen, E. W. (2008). Physical activity in the prevention and treatment of anxiety and depression. Nordic Journal of Psychiatry, 62(sup 47), 25–29.

[16] Josefsson, T., Lindwall, M., & Archer, T. (2014). Physical exercise intervention in depressive disorders: meta-analysis and systematic review. Scandinavian Journal of Medicine & Science in Sports, 24(2), 259–272.

[17] Schoenfeld, T. J., Rada, P., Pieruzzini, P. R., Hsueh, B., & Gould, E. (2013). Physical exercise prevents stress-induced activation of granule neurons and enhances local inhibitory mechanisms in the dentate gyrus. The Journal of Neuroscience, 33(18), 7770–7777.

[18] Oh, B., Butow, P., Mullan, B., Clarke, S., Beale, P., Pavlakis, N., & Rosenthal, D. (2010). Impact of medical Qigong on quality of life, fatigue, mood and inflammation in cancer patients: a randomized controlled trial. Annals of Oncology, 21(3), 608–614. doi: 10.1093/annonc/mdp479

[19] Chan, A. W., Lee, A., Suen, L. K., & Tam, W. W. (2011). Tai chi Qigong improves lung functions and activity tolerance in COPD clients: a single blind, randomized controlled trial. Complementary Therapies in Medicine, 19(1), 3–11. doi: 10.1016/j.ctim.2010.12.007

[20] Schmitz-Hübsch, T., Pyfer, D., Kielwein, K., Fimmers, R., Klockgether, T., & Wüllner, U. (2006). Qigong exercise for the symptoms of Parkinson's disease: a randomized, controlled pilot study. Movement Disorders, 21(4), 543–548.